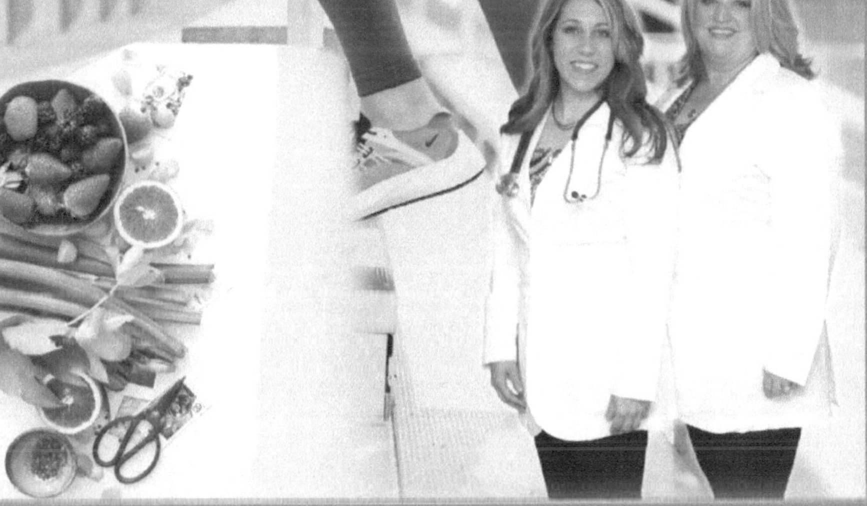

SUPERIOR
HEALTH & WELLNESS
DR. JODIE SCHULTZ   DR. JILL HOWE

Superior Health & Wellness of Gurnee

Providing Superior Health for our patients

Dr. Jill Howe & Dr. Jodie Schultz

Disclaimer

While the authors have used their best efforts in preparing this book, they make no representations or warranties with respect to accuracy or completeness of the contents of this book. The advice and strategies contained herein may not be suitable for your situation. You should consult a professional where appropriate. The authors shall not be liable for any loss of profit or any other special, incidental, consequential, or other damages. The purchaser or reader of this publication assumes responsibility for the use of these materials and information. Adherence to all applicable laws and regulations, both advertising and all other aspects of doing business in the United States or any other jurisdiction, is the sole responsibility of the purchaser or reader.

We Provide Superior Health
To Our Patients

Go to:
https://www.facebook.com/SuperiorHealthGurnee/

About the Authors

Dr. Jill Howe
& Dr. Jodie Schultz

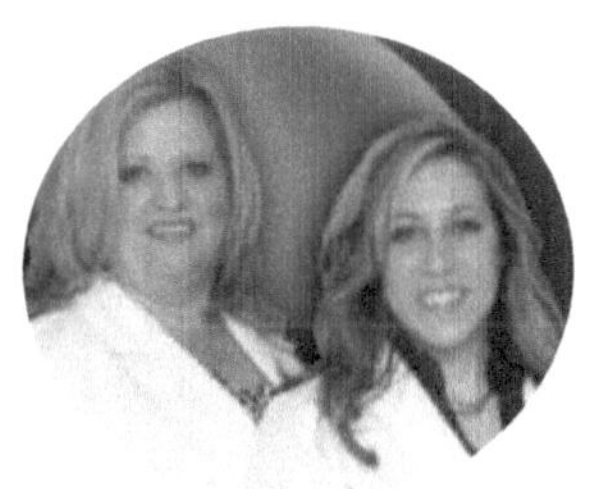

Dr. Jill Howe

I graduated from high school in 1983 was going to school to become an exercise physiologist. I soon realized I was basically going to be a glorified aerobics instructor and thought maybe I should pursue something a little bit different. My interests had always been in health, wellness and medicine, so I thought about becoming a heart surgeon.

While pursuing a degree in traditional medicine I attended an undergrad lecture about human function and human anatomy and the way the body is supposed to work. I was talking to one of my classmates and asked her how she was going to use this information. She told me she was going to become a chiropractor. I asked what chiropractors do because I thought they just worked on necks and backs.

She said, "Oh no. Let me tell you about all the different ways chiropractors can help because they work with the nervous system. They don't work with the neck. They work with the nerves that run through the neck and the places in the body that those nerves control."

I then began thinking about the significance of literally having someone's life in my hands as a heart surgeon. I realized there might be something I could do to prevent that from happening. That's when I decided to become a chiropractor.

During chiropractic school I learned the basics about human function and human anatomy and the way the body is supposed to work versus traditional medicine, which is more sick care and putting the body back together after it's broken. In chiropractic school I also learned a philosophy that helped me realize I was in the right place. There is something a lot more basic and fundamental and natural that can be done to help a body function properly and help a person not just get rid of symptoms but fix the reason that they have those symptoms.

I didn't want to have someone come to me with a headache and give them a pill to get rid of their headache. I wanted to be able to help the person with a headache know they had injured their neck and that we not only could help them with headaches but also prevent future problems for the injury to the nerves, neck, shoulders, arms and hands. I wanted to help them improve their overall health.

I've been in practice for over 20 years – it goes by so quickly. While I was in school, I realized I could make help people feel better without drugs or surgery if that was appropriate. But once I got into practice, I came into contact with the real world and with people's viewpoints on health, their considerations about what's okay and what's not okay for their body, what they're willing to do, what they're not willing to do.

I got the opportunity to interact with people in a way that was conversational. "What's going with you? How does that affect you?" More so, not just "where does it hurt" but "what's it like to be in your body for a day and what does it feel like and how do these problems negatively impact your life?" My favorite thing to do is to go out and educate patients because that is the definition of physician – an educator or a teacher. I really enjoy this because I get a chance to educate the average person who maybe treats their headaches with aspirin and doesn't know a different way. Not only can I educate them about what might be causing their headaches but that they can actually improve their health, not only their headaches but their whole body. They can sleep better; have more energy; get rid of sinus problems or jaw pain. It's all connected. To see them have their "A-ha" moment when I'm talking to them and when I'm educating them is really what validates everything that I've done up to this point.

The information I share during educational events is based on what I have learned in school but also through the work I've done with patients. My actual experience as a practicing chiropractor helping hundreds of people is what I bring to my lectures. I believe it best to bring actual experience vs. theoretical information in a book. I've learned to accommodate or adapt the way I treat each person based on their specific needs. I can't talk to person A the same way I talk to person B. The more I interact with people, the more it helps me when I go out and educate people that I've never met before. And that's the most exciting to me because they come thinking "I'm going to learn about a new pill or a new shot or a new surgery to help my carpal tunnel problems in my wrist" and then they learn "Really, it could be connected to the car accident I had when I was 16?" and to see them have that understanding and really get "Hey! Maybe something can be done about this" is so rewarding.

Dr. Jodie Schultz

When I was a junior in high school my horse got hurt by getting stuck in her stall and twisting around trying to get up. For months and months, we couldn't figure out what was wrong with her. She could barely walk and was deteriorating by the day. We had our vet out to check her out and he could never figure out what was wrong. He ran test after test and never found a solution to her problem. One day a massage therapist came out to the barn and my mom asked if there was anything she could do could help my horse. The lady said she could possibly help but before she touched my horse she wanted a chiropractor to see her. A vet who was an animal chiropractor came out to see her and Ran even more tests. He couldn't figure out what was wrong, so he told us he wanted the chiropractor who taught him to come out and look at her. So, a few days later the vet and chiropractor came and checked out my horse. they did all sorts of things on her that looked like voodoo and went on their way. They said they'd be back in the next day or so. The next day I get a call from one of the ladies at the barn and she tells me your horses feeling better and I asked what you mean? she said your horse is jumping the geese in the pasture. I said to her that's not possible because the day before she could hardly walk. Once I went and saw my horse and saw that this is true I thought to myself if this can help animals imagine what this could do for people.   It was then that I decided that I wanted to be a chiropractor.

I actually went to chiropractic school without ever getting adjusted. My first week of school I walked in the clinic and told them that I wanted to start getting adjusted. I was somebody who had suffered from chronic headaches. I had headaches every day and I was on medication to help prevent them. I have been told by my neurologist that I would always be on medication and if I went off it I would get headaches again. I was quickly referred to a chiropractor who had become a neurologist in the area and after seeing him he told me to continue to get adjusted and within three months had weaned me off all of my medications. I have been medication free for over 10 years now.

We always wanted to have a multidisciplinary practice. As chiropractic physicians we've integrated Eastern and Western medicine into our physical wellness center. This means we have chiropractors, medical doctors, physician assistants and nurse practitioners all working together for the betterment of our patients.

At our wellness center we offer spinal rehabilitation. We also work with nutrition; help to detoxify the body and we work diligently with our patients to help them regain their health. We don't work with their symptoms, we work with people to get their bodies functioning like they should be, so they don't have to constantly endure aches, pains and sickness. Instead they can just go and live the life that they're supposed to.

We've had the opportunity to lecture a great deal throughout our careers. Dr. Howe was invited to speak to chiropractic colleagues about digestive problems as well as a group of 400 doctors at a national convention. We've been asked to educate fire fighters and policemen and the general public at a variety of companies on topics like neuropathy (where the nerves are dying), fibromyalgia (where somebody feels like they have the flu all the time), neck and back pain.

We hosted a women's hormone symposium for 180 people and had multiple educators present. It was fantastic to hear from the audience what their struggles were and for them to realize there's something different that can be done about their problems.

There are two ways to read this book.

One:

If you are not affected by one of the conditions we describe in this book, chances are you know someone who is. You can skip to that chapter, read it and either then skip to the Epilogue, or give it to the person who it affects.

Or Two:

We hope you read the entire book start to finish, and then make sure you flow the directions in the Epilogue to make sure you take the next steps in putting the Three Step Superior Solution to work for you.

We have also added additional resources at the ends of some of the chapters – there are additional medical articles and references available for you to learn more about how the Three Step Superior Solution can get you the Superior results that other patients of ours have gotten.

If just one person's life is changed based on what we wrote here, then this book will have done our job.

Yours in Health,

Dr. Jill & Dr. Jodie

Contents

Chapter 1

Getting to Know
Dr. Jill & Dr. Jodie

1

About Jill

I was born and raised in Arlington Heights, Illinois. I went to the National College of Chiropractic in Lombard, Illinois. I always knew I wanted to be a doctor, but I thought I was going to be a heart surgeon until I learned more about natural health care and the fact that you don't have to wait until someone's life is literally in your hands to make a change for them. So, I went the direction of natural healthcare, and I became a chiropractic physician in 1989 and loved it ever since. And just the things that we've learned through our affiliations with other doctors and groups have helped us build a bigger, better practice, taught us other ways to help people, rather than just traditionally what you learn in school.

About Jodi

Sure. So, I grew up in Lindenhurst, Illinois, and I went to Antioch High School and then went to chiropractic. Well, actually I went to undergrad at the University of Kentucky, studied in Greece for a semester. Yep. And then went to Palmer College of Chiropractic in Davenport, Iowa, which then afterwards I moved back to the area and then had moved into Wisconsin but opened a practice in Illinois. So, I currently live in Kenosha, Wisconsin, right across the border. Practice obviously here in Illinois.

And honestly, when I went to college, I didn't necessarily know what I was going to do, but my horse got hurt. So, she got injured, and traditional veterinary medical care etc. didn't do anything and help. So ultimately, we had a chiropractor come out, and we were basically at the point we were going to have to put her down because she was just getting chronically worse. Could hardly walk, was losing hundreds of pounds of weight and a chiropractor did his voodoo because, at the time, that's what it was. I didn't know anything about it. And literally the next day, she was jumping the geese in our pasture. So, once the interference was removed from her body, she felt better and she was functioning.

And for me, it was kind of one of those things where I was like, "Wow if this can help animals, imagine what this could do for people." And so, I pretty much there kind of decided I was going to go to chiropractic school. I went to chiropractic school, the first week of school. I walked into the clinic because I had a chronic headache. They referred me to a neurologist, and this neurologist was a chiropractor before he became a neurologist, he started getting me adjusted, and within three months, my headaches went away. And as long as I'm aligned, I don't get headaches. So, it was definitely life-changing for me. And over time, what we do in our practice has evolved to help people in so many different ways. So that's how I got into it.

Studying in Greece

When I went to freshman orientation at the University of Kentucky, there was a professor who did one of our orientation classes, and he was really entertaining. And he was like, "Hey guys, I teach ancient mythology, and you have to take humanities anyways, you need two semesters of humanities, so take my class." And I was like, "All right." I liked him, so I took it. So, the first class was Greek mythology and the second one was the art of Greece and Rome. And I absolutely had no idea I loved that. And so, I was like, "Hey mom, I want to go study abroad in Greece," and she was on board with it. So, when I went to Greece, I went to the University of Indianapolis Athens campus, and I studied the Greek language, Greek art and archeology, Greek history and Greek philosophy.

So literally, all my requirements for chiropractic school were done. So, I got to just study the culture, and I lived with four other American students, but the program was small. There was like eight of us, and we were in an English school, but we literally took trips, part of the program was taking trips. My Greek art and archeology class, we went to the Parthenon and learned about it, we went to the ancient cemetery, we went to different ruins and we pretty much learned onsite, hands-on. And through that, I made friends at another school there called the American College of DEREE, and that was mostly Greek students going to an English school there. And I got ingrained in the culture and stayed with my friends, with their families who spoke Greek and not English. And I got to do Greek Easter. I mean, I went to all the different archeological sites and yeah, if I wasn't a chiropractor, I'd be an archeologist. It was cool. So, on spring break, we flew out to Rhodes and then we took boats to like eight different islands in seven days. And then we drove through the Peloponnesus and visited [inaudible 00:07:27] all the different sites. And then we also got to go up to the Thessaloniki and visit Delphi. And then I had friends who have property on Crete. And so, we got to go to the Palace of Knossos, and it was amazing.

What's the Big Motivation

Well, I just started looking more into it. I mean, I was in undergrad, I was studying premed, and I started talking to a friend who ended up being my roommate in chiropractic school. We were talking about why she said she wanted to be a chiropractor. And I said, "Well, what can you do with that?" And she started telling me about it, and I thought, "This is incredible, I can affect every part of the body, not just the heart. And I don't have to wait until people are dying and on the operating table for me to help them, I can intervene way before that." And so, I really decided right then and there, like, "Yeah, I'm going to check this out."

And it's really, at the school I went to, you're taught to think outside the box. It's not just about the spine and the nervous system, but the effect that it has on the entire body and how essential it is. It really spring-boarded me into all the things we do now in our practice. And there's just so many different things I never even thought we would be doing that we have the opportunity to help people with. Especially right now, like with the virus. We're doing testing and reaching out to companies and trying to keep the workforce safe and moving forward. And so, it's just, it's been amazing.

What are some treatments you provide?

Well, I feel like we have a holistic approach. So, someone will come in, and they have back pain, let's say, and we know everything's connected in the body. So we start looking at other areas only to find out they were a baseball catcher all through high school and college and their knees are bugging them and they have problems with their metabolism, or they have diabetes, or as Jodi said, they have headaches. And so, we really look at the entire person, and they're surprised when we tell them, "This is the plan we have, but all the things you talk to us about are going to start to improve." We see it time and time again.

And knowing how the body's going to improve, it gives us the confidence to keep people coming in even when they know, "I'm a little sore from what we did last time," we're able to educate them like, "That's a good thing. Here's what's happening." And to be able to provide them with the honest answers and the roadmap pretty much to regain their health is everything. It makes us feel not only confident but excited when people do get that relief, and they go, "Oh my gosh, I never thought I'd be headache free" or "I never thought that... Everyone in my family has this, and I don't have it anymore. That's so cool." So, everything from weight loss to back pain, to joint degeneration, to headaches, to breathing problems, hormone imbalances, food issues like food sensitivities, or I don't know, pretty much you name it.

We want to look at the whole chain, the whole person. And that's the beauty of the nervous system, because it doesn't just make the muscles work or allow you to feel or not feel pain, but it actually controls all the functions in your body. So, the same nerves that might go to muscles in your legs also control the function of digestive organs and glands. So we know, like when you have a heart attack, and you feel pain in your chest, but down your left arm or in your shoulder, if you just look at the shoulder, you might miss the cause of the problem, which could be your heart malfunctioning.

So, it is great to be able to put them together and to help people understand, because like you said, they come in having a bunch of different problems, and they feel like, "I'm falling apart, and I'm only 30." And then come to find out, they really are all interconnected. And once we start getting one working better, the rest of them fall into line, and it makes them feel confident and trust their body again.

The Approach We Take With Our Patients

Well, I think first and foremost, the thing that makes us different is that we're medically integrated. So, Jodi and I are both chiropractic physicians, but we have also gone to nursing school so that we could get a little bit more of the other side of, "Know what your competitors are going to do, know what's out there and what's offered." But at the time, we have a nurse practitioner, and we have a medical doctor. So, we have the best of both worlds combined. And so, it starts with the consultation with getting the person to see, "Hey, these headaches that you're having, when did they start?" "Well, they started around here." "Well, did anything happen around that time?" So, we delve into their past and don't just look at where does it hurt, and like you said, stick a shot there, or just focus on that.

So, getting the patient to really trust us and open up once they see that we're really invested in not just getting rid of their symptoms, but helping them regain their health and their function, that's where it starts. And then they start to open up about everything that's going on. And so many times I'll ask them, "Even if you didn't think it was connected, is there anything else going on?" Just because we understand the physiology, the function. So, if they say, "I have back pain," we'll ask them, "If you're a woman, do you have problems with your cycle? Do you have digestive issues? Do you have pain in your legs?" And so really helping them see how it is all connected. Then, our medical practitioner will take over and do a traditional medical exam. And then we get x-rays.

And so, it's really a lot of different types of training and a bunch of different eyes on that person. And then, we come up with a plan as a team on what that person needs. And then we educate them, so they understand, and they can make an informed decision. So, I don't say, "Sam, you have to do this." I tell you, as Jodi said with the headaches, "There's the bone pressing on a nerve that controls blood supply to your head. You can take all the aspirin you want, but that's not going to fix the cause of the problem. You're going to have to just keep treating the symptoms." So, once you, the patient sees, "Oh, really, all had to do is this type of treatment, and I can get it corrected?" Then I say, "The choice is yours. What do you want to do?" And I'm not telling them as the doctor, what they have to do. We're just sharing with them what the team has found and what we recommend.

Our team meets together and discusses the patient and discusses, "Hey, here's what I found. Here's what I see going on. Here's what their x-rays look like." So, the nurse practitioner is looking at that with us as the chiros going through all the orthopedics, talking about their history and what's going on. And we look at them as a whole. And so, we all look and go, "Hey, this, this, and this could help. This can help remove that. This can help get them out of pain." And then when we explain what's wrong, it's "Hey, here's what's going on, and here's what we can do to correct it."

So, we want the patient educated as well. And it's not just me saying, "Well, this is what I think you should do." It's collectively, "Well, our nurse practitioner and our chiros and our physical therapist all got together, and here's what they came up with literally together." So, it's not that, "Oh, you have to go down the street and get this piece done. And then you'll see your doctor five miles from here to look at this piece." It's really kind of one place where we can ideally take care of all of it.

What We Can Offer Our Patients

I think first and foremost; they need to understand the why, why is this problem happening, and what would you do about it? And then, "What's going to happen to me once you do that? What can I expect?" People will ask us; like "How soon do you think I'm going to start feeling better? How long is this going to really take?" And the coolest thing is legally you have to treat the patient and not their insurance. Some clinics don't do that. But I tell people when I give them their report on what the team has recommended, I already have, as Jodi said, I already have their x-rays, I already have all their exam findings, I have their insurance benefits, I know what insurance says they're going to cover. So, we estimate for them what their cost is going to be. There are no hidden fees. And I have no control over their insurance or what's needed for them.

But I tell them, "You don't have to like what I'm going to tell you, but I want you to understand it. And then you need to make an informed decision. So, it's not about money. It doesn't matter if it was free. If it doesn't make sense to you, if you don't feel like this is going to help you get the results you need and want, it doesn't matter." So, they really need to have trust. And they really need to know that that person feels confident in being able to help them. And when I say that person, I mean that office.

And also, a big thing as well, is people don't know to go in what the exam should look like. And so, a lot of people will come to us and be like, "Well, my doctor never took x-rays. That's a preference, but I don't have x-ray vision. So, I can't see what's going on inside. You can have a cavity and not have pain in your tooth, and that's the same thing with your spine. You can have underlying problems that we can't see or don't come out on the exam that x-rays are a really helpful tool. They're a big thing to let us know, like, what is your body already been through? What sort of breakdown are we seeing that can let us know what's going on?

And so, like a lot of people, we take x-rays on almost all of our patients. There are occasions where we don't need them, or they're not recommended, but for the most part, we're always doing that because we just don't have x-ray vision. So, I can't see what has happened over the last 30, 40, 50 years on the inside of you. And that's one piece that gives us that.

And we also use those to help show people the changes after they've gotten care as well. So, we tell them,

"So Sam, this is what your neck should look like. Here's where it is. After this much care, we're going to take another x-ray, and this is what we expect to see." So, I can show you proof that you've made the changes that you need to maintain your health.

It also helps us to keep them accountable because they can come in and tell us they're doing their exercises. And if we don't see the expected changes, we know they're not. So, we know how the process goes and what we should expect the findings to be. So, if they're doing what they should be doing, we should be getting certain results. And so, it helps us figure out if they are, or if we need to take a different approach as well.

The Biggest Misconception about Chiropractic?

Probably one of the biggest ones we always hear is like, "Oh, if I go to see them once, I have to go for the rest of my life." So we work from the standpoint of really trying to correct the underlying issues, but also give people tools that allow them to maintain it on their own. But at the same time, educating them about the type of stressors in their life and on their body that might... It would help them understand why they might consider making this a lifestyle choice. Whereas you go to the gym stay in shape, you go to the dentist every six months to keep your teeth functioning. So, your body's under a lot of stress. So why wouldn't you get adjusted every so often to undo that stress and to keep your body functioning as well as it can?

In my previous practice, we got into helping golfers. And it was talking about how your body is the most important piece of equipment that you have. It doesn't matter. Like Tiger Woods is an amazing golfer, but if he's got a back problem, he's not going to golf as well as he could. So that's 100% right. It is a software update.

And we, like Jodi said, one of the biggest things we do is tell people what to look for. If this is happening, like you might've thought headaches every day was normal, but now that you don't have them, when you start to get headaches or when you get rundown or if you're a woman and it's around the time of your cycle, or if you eat something that your body doesn't break down well, look for these symptoms. And these are things you can do in the real world to try to combat those symptoms. But if this happens, then you know, "Okay, it's time to come back in and get a couple of treatments." And so, people don't have to go once a week forever.

And then the other thing I was going to say is that one thing that we really have learned in our postgrad education, and I think this makes us extremely valuable is a way to actually make a lasting change in the body. So an adjustment is kind of similar to taking a pill. This is my opinion after 29 years in practice, it takes away the cause of the problem at the time. But if you want to really get a lasting change, you have to put in the rehab therapy that we do as well, because that's restructuring your body to handle the effects of gravity pushing down on you all day, every day.

Who is the most famous person you've ever treated?

So for me, it was Brian Urlacher. So my first two years in practice, the clinic I worked at, we were the official clinic for the Chicago Bears. So the Bears would come into the clinic, and my boss would go to games and Halas Hall and adjust them there. So there was a time he was gone, and I was covering for him, and Brian came in. And I'm a pretty small human being. I'm five feet tall, and I weigh 120 pounds. Brian Urlacher's thigh is as large as my torso. So, and I'm certified in some muscle work. I was doing it, and I had his thigh on my shoulder, and I was just like, "This is a very large human being."

He was very nice, super nice. All the bears' players were very nice. So yeah, we got to meet quite a few of them. So that was kind of fun.

Yeah. So that's when we were treating them. So my boss got to go to the Superbowl with them. And we showed up, Devin showed up for the first seven seconds of the game, caught the pass, scored and then they forgot to play the rest of the Superbowl. That was super fun.

Chapter 2

Achieving Optimal Health And Wellness

The definition of wellness according to the Merriam Webster dictionary is: the quality or state of being in good health especially as an actively sought goal. Likewise the definition of being healthy is: having good health: not being sick or injured. From that we can conclude that health and wellness is functioning at 100% or as close to it as possible, with every part of the body working properly. However, people frequently don't realize their health problem is not normal. People ignore their problems and mistakenly believe, "Everyone in my family has it" or "I'm just getting older" or "It will go away on its own" or even "It's from that high school injury that I had" and accept that the back pain, headaches, trouble sleeping, digestive issues and fatigue are normal.

Our society has learned to accept these things in part because others in the family have the same challenges or we've been raised to minimize our symptoms and just push through. But wellness is really about having the body functioning at 100% not just being symptom-free. Sometimes people forget what it's like to feel 100% and instead continue suffering quietly. It's heartbreaking when a patient comes in and tells us they have been suffering for 15 years.

We're one of the most technologically advanced nations and yet one of the sickest. The US spends more than 2.6 trillion dollars on healthcare per year, but we are only rated fifty-first in life expectancy worldwide. There seems to be some type of disconnect, why aren't we healthier? The truth is there are ways for people to be healthier if we're willing to get educated, take responsibility and make changes.

There is a video about a Gulf War paratrooper named Arthur who jumped out of planes so much that he sustained significant back and his knee injuries. Upon his release from the armed services Drs. told him that he should accept that he would never walk normally again and at a certain point Arthur just accepted that. His inability to walk without experiencing significant pain led to inactivity and weight gain. He continued to deteriorate and eventually had to rely on crutches or a wheelchair to support himself for his daily activities. This video documented Arthur's journey from nearly being an invalid (who because of rapidly declining health had accepted that he would soon die) to somebody who is now not only able to stand unassisted and move about his home but is capable of running. He was convinced because of the prognosis the Drs. gave him that he would never walk again. Don't let anyone tell you that you can't, that you're done because if you not only want and believe you can do something but are willing to take action then you can achieve your health goals.

Another big challenge with healthcare is insurance companies. People often forget insurance companies are a business and their goal are to make money, not get you healthy. Insurance companies have guidelines of what healthcare is. To them, healthcare is minimizing symptoms to a certain degree. Patients come in and they want to get care based on what their insurance company covers, however, that may not include the type of care that best addresses their specific health problem. The insurance company covers certain procedures, however, the Dr's. job is to evaluate and treat the patient standing in front of them without regard to the insurance card that the patient carries. It's likely that an insurance company will approve a treatment that is more "cost effective" (medication for a headache) versus one that is aimed at correcting the actual cause of the problem. We've never seen anyone have a headache due to an aspirin deficiency. True healthcare should be delivered based on the most effective form of treatment, not the least expensive. It would be like telling someone with cancer I have a cure for you and having them say their insurance company doesn't cover it, so they continue to suffer. It really comes down to helping the patient understand the difference between health and what their insurance will cover.

Our philosophy is to help patients understand how we can help them by addressing the cause of their problem and not just the symptom. We're dedicated to educating the patient so they understand the exact cause of their health concern so they can make the most informed decision about the treatment that's right for them. It is their body, so in the end it's up to that individual to make the best choice for themselves.

We aren't looking to help patients be just symptom-free but rather function at their highest possible level. The body must lose over 60% function in an area in order to experience a symptom. The same is true with your car, when your oil light goes on it doesn't mean you're just a quart low, it goes on when it's at a level that is dangerous if you continue to ignore it. The same is true with symptoms, when you get a symptom, your body has been dealing with the cause of that problem for a long time. So, when a symptom goes away and a patient tells us they're "better" we perform a re-evaluation to determine if the cause of the problem has been resolved, not just the symptoms.

If a floor tile in your house was loose and cracked and you think, "I have another one. I'm just going to put that tile down" you may come to find out that the foundation under the tile is causing the cracked tile because it's uneven. So, what it looks like on the surface has nothing to do with what's really causing the problem. Sure, you could replace the tile in your house but then the rest of the floor will continue to buckle and break and down the road it's going to end up costing more money. The same is true with your health. When you just treat symptoms, you allow the underlying cause of the problem to continue and it gets worse. We address the cause of the problem, not just the symptoms.

Chapter 3

Headaches

Headaches are quite common. Someone gets a headache and then takes an aspirin or Tylenol. But there are many different reasons why a person has a headache including: lack of sleep; eye strain; staying up too late; skipping meals; a sinus infection; following a car accident or even a brain tumor. If a person takes an aspirin, they don't really know what it is they are treating. The aspirin just increases blood flow to the brain, but they are not fixing the cause of the problem. Unless the real cause is addressed, the symptom will continue to return, or the problem will get worse.

Most people are unaware that only two headaches a year are considered normal. Two headaches a year is normal and more than that, your body is trying to tell you something.

If your car didn't start you wouldn't just think it will probably start tomorrow or just hitch a ride with a friend. You would wonder what is going on and take it to the mechanic. Our society takes better care of our cars than we do of our bodies. We can get a new car, we can't get a new body, yet.

Your medical doctor may not consider four headaches in the past four months a serious problem (unless they were migraines). If these headaches are yours, you know how annoying they are. You know how they make it hard to do your job, enjoy you hobbies, let alone perform your normal daily routine. This is a serious problem that needs to be addressed.

Maybe your experience has gone something like a current patient of ours: you go to the Dr. to find out why you're having headaches. They spend a total of five minutes talking to you after which time they prescribe a medication and schedule a follow-up appointment in one month. A month later you return to tell them the medication isn't working. At that time, they recommend another, more powerful drug to control your headaches and hope next month they'll be handled. At your second month follow-up appointment when you tell them you're still suffering, they send you for further testing to rule out any serious causes of your headaches (brain tumor, cancer, etc.) When your tests return negative then they may recommend a third medication. If upon your fourth visits the headaches are not under control, you may have told there's nothing else they can do, and you just have to live with it.

There is a philosophical difference between health care and sick care. Sick care is symptom-based treatment. Patients go to a doctor because something hurts. The doctor tells them to take some medication and then let them know how they're feeling. Or maybe the patient has a rash that has been developing for a week. The doctor might give them a cream to use and see what happens. They're treating just the symptoms. Healthcare involves getting to the root of the problem and developing a treatment program to correct that cause.

The nervous system controls everything in the body - every organ, every muscle and every gland. It allows you to feel hot or cold, pain, the position of your body in space, it controls the beating of your heart and your ability to breathe along with digesting your food and nourishing all the cells in your body. Any interruption of this communication results in malfunctioning of the area supplied by those nerves. If you walk into your house and all the lights were on and all of a sudden, they all went out. You wouldn't go to each room and flip on and off the light switch or change the light bulbs in each room. You would go to the fuse box. You would go to the thing that supplies the power to the house.

So, in our office we go to the power supply of the body which is the nervous system. Our examination focuses on the nervous system and the spine that surrounds and protects it. By doing that, we're able to assess the function of the nerves and the area(s) they control. This allows us to determine the source of the problem and often times find additional problems before they manifest symptoms. For instance, pressure on the nerves that control blood supply to the head can result in light headedness, dizziness and headaches, but also because of their anatomical position in the neck a person may experience ear infections, neck pain or trouble with their vision. Patients appreciate that because we'll work them up and they'll say, "I came for headaches." In our work up we may find other problem areas the patient was unaware of due to the severity of their headaches.

All good doctors know the importance of getting an accurate diagnosis of a patient's problem. But why is this so important? It's important because without knowing what the disease or injury is, the treatment cannot be directed to the actual problem.

Unfortunately, when it comes to headaches, many patients do not receive an accurate diagnosis. If a patient were to see a doctor with a pain in the head and the doctor were to conclude that you have a pain in your head (headache), this tells little about the actual problem. In headache patients, we've become very good at labeling problems-giving them a name. If the headache comes and goes, we call it episodic. If it occurs suddenly, we call it acute, and if it occurs over many years we say it is chronic. But are these labels really helpful?

The reality is everyday people show up in doctors' offices, obtain cursory examinations and walk out with a prescription for their head pain. Not all doctors do this, of course, but with the time constraints of managed care and the insurance company oversight, a doctor's visit is just not what it used to be. When was the last time you had a house call from a doctor? Of course, the worst case is when a patient acts as their own doctor, sees an advertisement for a pill and does the diagnosing himself or herself!

In chiropractic, we may also label your headache as tension-type, migraine or chronic, but a good chiropractor will not stop there. The label does not give much of an indication of what needs to be done, and more importantly we still do not know the CAUSE of the pain. Clinical experience and research over many decades have shown that many headaches are actually caused by injuries to the neck and spine. But if a doctor does not examine the neck, they may not discover these hidden injuries. Sometimes an astute doctor will take a history and it may be discovered you had a whiplash or other neck trauma, months or even years earlier. This is important information to get at the cause.

We take a comprehensive approach to headache patients at our clinic. A detailed history about the location, duration, and quality of pain is followed up by a thorough physical examination, especially of your spinal column. We may also order imaging tests such as x-rays to see the positions of the individual vertebrae in your neck.

Patients ask us if this approach is so successful, "Why doesn't my doctor do this?" This could be for two reasons. First, the philosophy of mainstream medicine focuses on the evaluation and treatment of symptoms. They're trained more for emergency and sick care. Secondly when patients ignore their problems and they get too bad, patients demand a quick fix. They're not interested in how they got this way; they just want to feel better now. Whereas, any doctor would prefer to help a person intervene before their symptoms become severe, there's a difference in philosophy on the most effective way to correct the problem.

Our office is a wellness center where we help patients by assisting the body's natural functions rather than putting them on medications. That's what makes Superior Health and Wellness unique. We focus on the patient as a whole instead of just a symptom or body part.

Have you ever stopped and wondered, "…which type of doctor should I go to for treatment of my headaches?" In order to make an informed decision, it is appropriate to look at the side effects each treatment option carries and then consider the pros and cons of each treatment.

It has been reported that 45 million Americans suffer from headaches, many on a daily basis. Though some just put up with the pain, others become totally disabled during the headache. Most people initially turn to an over the counter drug such as a non-steroidal anti-inflammatory drug (NSAID) of which there are 3 types: 1) salicylates, such as aspirin; 2) traditional NSAIDs, such as Advil (ibuprofen), Aleve (naproxen); and, 3) COX-2 selective inhibitors, such as Celebrex.

According to the medical review board of About.com, complications of NSAID drugs include stomach irritation (gastritis, ulcer), bleeding tendencies, kidney failure, and liver dysfunction. Some NSAIDs (particularly indomethacin) can interfere with other medications used to control high blood pressure and cardiac failure and long-term use of NSAIDs may actually hasten joint cartilage loss, leading to premature arthritis. Another over the counter commonly used drug is Tylenol (Acetaminophen) in which liver toxicity can be a potential side effect (particularly with long term use).

Here's the kicker – only about 60% of patients respond to a 3-week trial of an NSAID, NSAIDs can mask signs and symptoms of infection, it cannot be predicted which NSAID will work best, and no single NSAID has been proven to be superior over others for pain relief. Moreover, estimates of death associated with NSAID (mostly gastrointestinal causes) range between 3200 on the low side to higher than 16,500 deaths per year in the United States. Another BIG concern is that low daily doses of aspirin, "…clearly have the potential to cause GI injury as 10mg of aspirin daily causes gastric ulcers."

Others may turn to prescription medication for hopeful pain relief. One of the more frequently prescribed medications for headaches is amitriptyline (commonly known as Elavil, Endep, or Amitrol). This is actually an antidepressant but was found to work quite well for some headache sufferers. The potential side effects include blurred vision, change in sexual desire or ability, constipation or diarrhea, dizziness, drowsiness, dry mouth, headache (ironically), appetite loss, nausea, tiredness, trouble sleeping, tremors and weakness. Allergic reactions such as rash, hives, itching, difficulty breathing, tightness in the chest, swelling of the mouth, face, lips or tongue, chest pain, rapid and/or irregular heart rate, confusion, delusions, suicidal thoughts or actions AND MORE are reported.

The pros and cons of chiropractic include a report on children under 3 years of age, where only one reaction for every 749 adjustments (manipulations) occurred (it was crying, NO serious side effects were reported). In adults, transient soreness may occur. Though stroke has been reported as a cause of headache, it was concluded that stroke "...is a very rare event...", and that, "...we found no evidence of excess risk of VBA stroke associated chiropractic care compared to primary care." Another convincing study reported that chiropractic was 57% more effective than drug therapy in reducing headache and migraine pain! They concluded – chiropractic first, drugs second and surgery last.

What about those drugs? Could the drugs you are on be causing your headaches?

According to the medical review board of About.com, complications of NSAID drugs include stomach irritation (gastritis, ulcer), bleeding tendencies, kidney failure, and liver dysfunction.

Some NSAIDs (particularly indomethacin) can interfere with other medications used to control high blood pressure and cardiac failure and long-term use of NSAIDs may actually hasten joint cartilage loss, leading to premature arthritis.

Another over the counter commonly used drug is Tylenol (Acetaminophen) in which liver toxicity can be a potential side effect (particularly with long term use).

What if you are taking prescription medication for your headaches?

One of the more frequently prescribed medications for headaches is amitriptyline (commonly known as Elavil, Endep, or Amitrol).

This is actually an antidepressant but was found to work quite well for some headache sufferers.

The potential side effects include blurred vision, change in sexual desire or ability, constipation or diarrhea, dizziness, drowsiness, dry mouth, headache (ironically), appetite loss, nausea, tiredness, trouble sleeping, tremors and weakness.

Allergic reactions such as rash, hives, itching, difficulty breathing, tightness in the chest, swelling of the mouth, face, lips or tongue, chest pain, rapid and/or irregular heart rate, confusion, delusions, suicidal thoughts or actions AND MORE are reported.

Wow! That sounds worse than the headache you had in the first place!

So what are the side effects of chiropractic care?

The pros and cons of chiropractic include a report on children under 3 years of age, where only one reaction for every 749 adjustments (manipulations) occurred (it was crying, NO serious side effects were reported).

In adults, transient soreness may occur.

Another convincing study reported that chiropractic was 57% more effective than drug therapy in reducing headache and migraine pain!

So how does the actual chiropractic treatment work?

Headaches are a common complaint at chiropractic clinics. There are many causes of headaches, some of which are "idiopathic" or, unknown. Some headaches arise from "vascular" (blood vessels) causes such as migraine and cluster headaches.   These often include nausea and/or vomiting and can be quite disabling and require rest in a dark, quiet place sometimes for a half or a whole day. Another type of headaches can be categorized as "tension" headaches.   These usually result from tightness in the muscles in the neck and upper back caused from stress, work, lack of sleep, sinusitis, trauma such as whiplash, and others.

So "how does chiropractic work?" To answer this, let's first discuss what we do when the headache patient comes in. First, the history is very important! Here, we'll ask "how/when did the headaches start. This may glean the actual cause of headaches such as a car accident or injury of some sort.

Next, we'll ask about activities that increase or create the headache, which gives us ideas of how we might help manage the headache patient. For example, when certain activities precipitate the onset of a headache, we will modify the workstation and/or give specific exercises on a regular schedule to keep the neck tension under control. When information gathered about what decreases or helps the neck pain and headaches, we will recommend treatments often that can be done at home such as a home traction unit. This would be suggested if we are told that "…pulling on my neck feels great!" The quality of pain (throbbing = vascular, ache and tightness = neck), intensity of pain (0-10 pain scale), and timing (worse in the morning vs. evening) help us track change after treatment is rendered, usually gathered once a month.

The examination includes blood pressure which can in itself create headaches when high, looking in the eyes to view the blood vessels in the back of the eye to make sure there is no evidence of increased pressure against the brain, ears – to see if there is an infection or wax blockage. This can help if there is dizziness and/or balance loss. We will sometimes listen to the throat as well as the heart to see if there may be a blockage, a valve problem, or other issues. Neck muscle tightness (spasm) will be evaluated along with the range of motion, paying particular attention to the positions/directions that increases and decreases pain, especially those that decrease pain. Nerve function by checking reflexes, sensation and muscle strength as well as correlating information like positions that decrease arm or leg pain will be included as any position that reduces pain in the arm or leg must be incorporated into an exercise. X-rays may include bending "stress" views so that ligaments (that hold bones together) can be evaluated for "laxity" (torn and unstable). When this is found, we avoid adjustments to these vertebrae.

As you can see, if is very important do a thorough evaluation so headache patients can be properly managed. Treatment approaches include: 1. Adjustments; 2. Soft tissue therapy (trigger point stimulation, myofascial release); 3. Posture correction exercises and other exercises; 4. Education about job modifications; 5. Co-management with other health care providers, if medication or injection therapy is needed.

If a person has headaches, they could go on a medication but that doesn't really fix the reason for the headaches. At our clinic, we want to know why a patient has a health problem.

For instance, when Walter Payton was diagnosed with liver cancer, Dr. Howe actually wrote him a letter that said you can absolutely get a liver transplant but there are nerves that control the function of that area of your body and it's essential that they work in order to fully heal. He was a well-known football player, and as great as he was, he still was subjected to a lot of physical traumas. Dr. Howe wanted the family to know that regardless of whether or not he got the transplant, we need to make sure that his body was working to the best of its ability.

We had a patient come in and Dr. Howe did a workup on her. She had neck and upper back pain and some shoulder pain. She stated in passing that every time she took a deep breath she experienced a stabbing pain in her back. I pushed right on part of her rib and she said, "Oh my gosh! That's the pain." Through our exam, we found out that her rib was slightly misaligned. It wasn't lined up exactly with the bones of the spine. A very simple treatment relieved what she had been suffering with for a year and a half.

Dr. Howe's best friend is an osteopathic physician and they go back and forth on treating with medicine and treating naturally but when she's in pain, Dr. Howe has been able to resolve symptoms faster using Physical medicine than the medication the Dr. was used to taking for these problems. The Dr. is always amazed and appreciative of the speed and thoroughness of her care.

Patients get the best results when they are proactive. They have to seek out the help and look for a better solution for what they're suffering with today. So it's really key to be proactive. When patients come to our center it's our job to educate them and help them understand the important role they must play to be part of the solution to their health problem. Otherwise, they are contributing to the cause of the problem. Our goal isn't to have people in the clinic all the time but rather to have them be a part of the healing process and teach them how to maintain a healthy lifestyle once they achieve it..

Chapter 4

Sick & Tired Of Being Sick & Tired

If you watch the news or read a newspaper you've already heard that health in America is declining. As a nation we're so technologically advanced that we can sit on our rear end and do almost anything. We can make a phone call, go to work or watch TV – and we never have to leave the comfort of our couch. Unfortunately, with all these conveniences we're becoming more and more sedentary and the quality of the food we eat is becoming less nutrient-rich resulting in increasing health problems and expanding waistlines.

This generation has developed technology to have our food ready, pay bills or even make a purchase at the touch of a button. As a result, people in our society are looking for things that are fast, even when it comes to healthcare. Americans demand results– "I want to feel better yesterday." "I can't miss any work." "I'm getting married in two weeks, I need to lose 20 pounds." So, we take things that we think are going to help us get to our goal. But we don't understand the reason we have the problem. Take headaches for example. When most people have a headache, they reach for a pain reliever. The true cause of their headache is not addressed by this type of medication; headaches are not caused by an aspirin deficiency.

All food, drinks and medication have to be detoxified through the liver. The liver is like a water treatment plant removing waste and harmful chemicals from the body to prevent damage to our cells. Our body comes into contact with chemicals on a daily basis (pesticides, food dyes, car exhaust and pollution, etc.). The more chemicals the liver has to process the less it can handle its normal day-to-day activities.

Many patients who come to our office tell us that they've "tried" several other doctors who weren't able to get them the results they expected. Throughout their search the problem is continually progressing making it more challenging to resolve. The longer a problem exists the more strain it places on the rest of the body. This is called compensation. The longer the body is allowed to malfunction, the more it compensates placing additional strain on the other systems.

As a Physical Medicine center, our philosophy is to engage the body's natural ability to heal. We don't utilize medication as a first line of treatment in our clinic as they don't address the cause of many health problems. There is a time and place for drugs in treating health problems. When a patient presents with headaches (as previously discussed), our goal is not only to get them relief as quickly as possible, but also get to the cause of the headaches so they don't have to rely on medication or whatever it is that's gotten them by up to this point.

The average senior citizen gets fifteen different prescriptions a year per the Journal of the American Medical Association 1992. This often includes high blood pressure medication. While medication can lower blood pressure, it often doesn't treat the reason for the elevation. According to the Mayo clinic, lifestyle changes including diet modification and exercise go a long way toward controlling high blood pressure. We're by no means suggesting anyone discontinue their medication without first consulting their physician as they have had the opportunity to fully evaluate your unique health concerns. However, it cannot be ignored that a diet rich in green leafy vegetables (spinach and arugula), low carbohydrate fruits (apples and pears) and lean protein (fish and chicken) that is also low in red meat (beef and pork), processed foods (potato chips and french fries), salt and sugar provides the body with the building blocks needed for faster repair and healing.

If a patient is put on high blood pressure (hypertension) medication but isn't educated about the connection between hypertension and diet the patient isn't going to change their eating habits. It's not uncommon for a patient with hypertension to also have elevated cholesterol. It's possible they're going to take a cholesterol medication which has Neuropathy as a potential side effect. This is because cholesterol medication reduces all forms of cholesterol in the body, even that which covers and protects our nerves. When the covering of the nerves becomes degraded it causes damage to the nerves. So, while the medication is targeting their heart and blood vessels, it's damaging their nerves. As a result of the nerve damage they can't feel their feet, so they get put on another medication for that symptom. It just keeps going and going because all these medications have side effects and put stress on the liver which results in more inflammation in the body. This inflammation puts more stress on the heart which drives up blood pressure, cholesterol and the decline in the patient's health snowballs from there.

Determining the reason a patient has their symptoms is like finding a needle in a haystack. The question is, why are you having the underlying problem? With elevated cholesterol, blood pressure, neuropathy and diabetes, what really is the underlying problem in the body? To us, helping a patient understand why they have their health problem is the most exciting part of what we do.

When you pay into an insurance plan each month, you expect to be able to utilize its benefits when seeking healthcare. Some people don't have insurance, have poor insurance or high deductibles and co-pays. What people don't realize is that insurance companies are businesses designed to make a profit at the end of the year. The more money they dispense to healthcare providers the less money they retain as profit. Therefore, insurance was designed to cover "sick care" (surgeries, medications, etc.) and not true healthcare which would be services or procedures that are preventative in nature.

This often results in patients neglecting their health because they can't afford treatment. Patients have shared stories of cutting their pills in half to make them last longer, foregoing non-covered medically necessary treatments or have lived with the burden of having to file bankruptcy due to medical expenses despite utilizing their insurance. That's unfortunate because the symptoms continue to exist and progress without necessary medical intervention and this is one of the reasons that the United States is one of the sickest countries but yet one of the most technologically advanced.

This is a big reason why we offer free workshops in our communities. Hopefully people can get some piece of information that will benefit them. We can't fix somebody with words, but we can give them information. Anybody can change their diet, drink more water or start walking. All those actions offset some of the negative stressors (pollution, poor diet and medication side effects, etc.) the patient experiences on a daily basis, however, without a treatment designed to address the true source of their health problems, their progress will plateau. We strive to make our services affordable and realistic for patients so they can be responsible and take charge of their health instead of allowing issues to escalate.

Many patients determine the route of treatment they'll pursue based on "what their insurance will pay for", allowing insurance companies to manage their healthcare, not doctors and other health practitioners who are board-certified to do so. It can be a challenge to convey the issues and nuances of a patient interaction to an insurance company. It's difficult to communicate in writing or doctors don't have an opportunity to spend a half an hour writing a dissertation on what happened with the patient. So, it's up to us, through our diagnosis, exam and treatment codes, to help paint a picture for the insurance company of what is going on with the patient. But the bottom-line is we're the doctors that are actually seeing that patient. We are examining them. We are interacting with them. We're observing whatever is going on with their health problem and hopefully being part of that solution. It may come down to dollars and cents for the insurance companies, and they have to have policies, but we believe there are many doctors who are in disagreement with some of the restrictions on policies in insurances. When medical professionals aren't able to offer a workable solution a patient often walks away thinking their health problems are age or genetic related and they "just have to live with it".

One of these "untreatable" conditions is called neuropathy. This occurs when the nerves, usually in the hands and feet, are deprived of oxygen and start to die. This is commonly found in people with diabetes and those who have survived cancer. They no longer have cancer but now they're left with this problem and many times because it's not really something the medical community treats very effectively; they prescribe medication that doesn't change the problem but alters the way in which patients perceive the discomfort they are in. This medication doesn't fix the nerves.

If somebody was choking you, you couldn't take a pill and make them stop choking you. They would physically have to take their hands off you and then you could breathe. The same is true with the nerves they require oxygen which isn't the purpose of Neuropathy medication; they're designed to block pain. We see many patients and they often ask us why we believe we can help them when their doctor couldn't. They think it's something they will have to live with. Every Dr. has their own specialty and if your Dr. wasn't trained specifically on your health problem, they won't have a workable solution.

Part of helping patients regain their health involves educating them that just because someone else in their family has a problem like headaches doesn't mean that their headaches have the exact same cause. The possible causes of headaches include (but are not limited to) car accidents, sinus infections, eye strain, food sensitivity, skipping meals, trauma or a brain tumor. The true cause of your health problem must be determined in order to provide an accurate solution.

Sometimes patients come to our clinic and will tell us their problems are genetic. "I have genetic back pain" or "I have genetic weight problems," or "I have genetic" something that I've never heard of. "I have genetic fibromyalgia."

Perhaps they've misunderstood something a doctor might have said such as, "you were genetically predisposed to have this problem" meaning you have higher cholesterol in your body and so your metabolism is slower. So therefore, you can't get rid of toxins and poisons and they build up in your system faster and that's what's giving you these fibromyalgia symptoms.

In our clinics we've had several patients come to us who could "not get better" in other places or had "genetic problems" and after applying the principles we use in our office their problem has been eliminated. And so we don't want people to think for one second that there is absolutely nothing that can be done about their problem. Look again. Be willing to look again because it is the only way it's going to get any better.

At our wellness centers we strive to communicate well with our patients, so they understand what is going on with their body. As doctors we were taught in medical school to run through the list of symptoms and figure out what's wrong. But really the consultation with the patient is all about getting the patient to understand that they have a problem. The examination and diagnostic testing help us determine the cause of the problem. We provide a thorough Report of Findings, so our patients fully understand what is causing their health problem, what the solution to their health concern is and our expectations for their care. This knowledge empowers them to make a difference in and take responsibility for their own health and life.

Even though we don't utilize traditional medication in our offices, it's our job, and part of our training, to know what these drugs do to the body and educate the patient by telling them that once their body starts functioning better, they may notice their medication working differently. We then refer them back to their prescribing doctor to make any necessary changes. When the body works as it's intended to, it doesn't require medication.

A particular patient came in who had undergone a significant number of tests and he was told that he was going to die. He said, "I had an MRI of my back. I had pain in my rear end and the pain went down in my leg and nobody can figure out what the problem is. My walking has been getting worse." Doctors were obviously looking for big things like multiple sclerosis or disc problems. This man's doctors and the hospitals had done literally $10,000 to $12,000 worth of testing.

Our evaluation of the patient revealed significant muscle spasms and restriction in the movement of his spinal joints. During the examination he said, "My gosh! That's the problem right there" and we were able to identify it. Testing does not get you healthy, it's about finding the cause as fast as possible so you can start making changes for the person.

We had another patient with a jaw problem called TMJ. She had spent a week in the hospital and couldn't open her mouth more than the size of a drinking straw. She was in so much pain and all she could eat was liquids. She came in and we did a workup on her and found she had a problem with her neck. We did a very simple technique on her jaw and she was so shocked that in a matter of minutes she could get so much relief where she had previously spent an entire week in the hospital. By the time she left our office after her first visit she was able to open her mouth the size of a medium-sized Dixie cup.

So that's really our niche – understanding how the body functions. Every doctor understands how the body works but understanding the importance of the entire body, not just the heart (like a Cardiologist) or just the glands (like an Endocrinologist) or just the joints (like an Orthopedist) but understanding how the whole body works together and using that knowledge to educate people and find solutions for them. We're not looking to cure high blood pressure or cancer but within the bounds of what we do, we are experts at healing problems that traditional medicine often can't correct.

For instance, with neuropathy, we have had people come in and their legs and feet are blue because they're not getting proper blood supply and they're not getting proper blood and nerve supply down to their feet. When they come in, we talk to them about different options like metabolism or rehabilitation if their body is not working properly. We educate them about what they are putting into their body that provides it with the nutrients it needs to either heal or create more problems in their system. We can help put some of the responsibility back on the patient for something like neuropathy when all they've been given is a pill before that didn't work because that's what doctors are being told is going to minimize the symptoms or cover up the symptoms so the patient doesn't have them because that's usually why we go to the doctor.

Being willing to go the distance with our patients, give them some tough love and educate is what's going to help. We let them know that we're not going to let reasons they are telling us as to why they can't get healthy get in their way. But in the end, it is always up to the patient. We can only take them so far.

As we have shared, we're not looking to cure cancer or high blood pressure but taking a pill isn't curing it either. We had a patient who came to us from Wisconsin and she had pancreatic cancer. It's very serious and very aggressive. Being from Wisconsin she consumed quite a bit of dairy. Every meal had dairy in some form. After providing a workup on her we suggested she take dairy out of her diet, not calcium but dairy and she did. Pancreatic cancer usually is so aggressive that people usually die within a couple of months, but we were able to extend her life span over two years. She made changes to her body and had improved her health to the point where she didn't want chemo, she didn't want radiation or anything like that. She improved the health of her body so much by just making a simple change like not putting something in that was creating stress on her body and she would have never known that because it was her favorite food.

There are some common health problems we find when working with upper, mid, and lower back. **W**e look at the spine and the nervous system and we incorporate traditional medical practitioners in a non-traditional way. They help us affect the changes in the areas of the body – the upper body meaning the neck and the shoulders, the middle back and the ribs and the spine in the middle back, and the lower body, the lower back and the hips and the tail bone.

There are 26 pairs of nerves in the body that come off the spinal cord. The spinal cord comes off the brain (right through the first bone in the neck and ultimately the nerves end down at the tailbone). Different injuries to those areas of the body will produce different symptoms, different health problems. By helping a person to understand it's not just headaches but rather looking at how their body handles blood flow to their head. The nerves controlling blood supply to the head are in the neck. We then explore the neck and ask if they have had any slips or falls or accidents. Are they on a computer all the time, and if so, in what position do they sit? We are looking to identify what is contributing to the problem. What might be injuring their neck?

Things like poor posture or carrying a child all the time can cause the middle back to have somewhat of a curve in it. Are you a woman carrying a big heavy purse on one side all the time? What are the challenges that different parts of the body face? Each nerve originates from the spinal core, leaves the spine and ends up in a specific area of the body (like the hands or feet). We look at the area of the symptom and then we backtrack to the spine to find out if there has been any damage or trauma to that area.

We have had people come in and we can see a big wallet in their back pocket, and we tell them they might want to put that in their front pocket. They often respond, "Yeah, yeah. My doctors already told me about that." When we simulate what happens to their body as a result of this they understand how their wallet placement is contributing to their sciatica. We're not saying model perfect posture is required all the time, but if patients understand and are thinking about how they can minimize stress on their body they can minimize damage to their nerves and spine. When patients can personally reduce the physical stresses on their body they can predict a much healthier future for themselves and, to some degree, reverse health problems they may have right now. Making small changes for themselves, patients can decrease the severity of their symptoms, the frequency of their symptoms, or even prevent a problem.

Simple things can help on a daily basis. Setting up things in the daily environment to support your back can help like a good chair at your desk, a supportive mattress in bed, and the position of your seat in the car. We had a patient who had rented a car that had a cockeyed driver's seat. When they got in just sitting in the seat hurt their back so much that they couldn't drive the car. They had to take it back and get a different vehicle.

We've gone into businesses and done an ergonomic study and made sure that employee workstations were supportive to the body. We've walked through Wal-Mart before, as a courtesy, and pointed out some potential places patrons or employees might injure themselves. If more companies understood the significance of subtle things, they could do to help improve the health of their employees this could significantly reduce their Worker's Compensation claims. We once wrote a prescription for a patient to get a new car. Her company gave her a car for her work that didn't fit her properly and it was causing more symptoms for her.

Many workplaces reward their teams with food, often foods with low nutritional value. Unfortunately, in this country, we are trained to go with what tastes good so extra sugar and flavor enhancers are added into foods, so we like those things better than the natural things. The more we have those processed foods the less our body responds to the natural tastes of things like carrots or something healthy like an apple. The cookies, donuts or muffins may be tasty but later in the day employees get sleepy. They're all falling asleep. None of them are paying attention at meetings. They are screwing up things in the office. If employers really looked at the production that they got out of the food they put in their employees, they might change their mind.

At our clinics we do a lot of work with patients on nutrition and changing people's diets. At the holidays instead of bringing us these wonderful cookies that they made, clients bring us big giant baskets of vegetables and fruits. It's just a matter of changing your mind and realizing it will catch up with you one day.

It's important to ask oneself just how much a health problem is bothering you. How much it is interfering with your life and then decide when you are ready to make a change. At that point in time hopefully your healthy decision will result in a better quality of life for you as well as rub off on the rest of the people in your life.

Chapter 5

Sports, Work & Automobile Related Accidents & Injuries

Accidents and injuries are common and often don't seem to cause damage to our body. What may seem like a minor injury can come back to haunt you and significantly affect your health down the line. If you've ever been in a car accident, it's essential to get your body evaluated, just like you would get your car checked out and repaired. The body goes through the exact same trauma that the car went through. However, our bodies aren't made of steel, are not as big as a car and are not designed to withstand that kind of impact.

Everybody seems to know that car accidents often cause whiplash and most people don't think it's a really big deal, but it can get worse over time. Whiplash can be caused by anything that jolts a person. This includes car accidents, sports hits, or even slips and falls. When whiplash occurs the muscles, tendons and ligaments that hold the head and neck in place are injured. This can lead to muscle spasm and pain and long-term instability in the neck. The whipping motion that happens to the spine has negative effects not only on the muscles but, even more importantly, on the spinal cord itself because it controls every other function in the body. You might not have back pain right after the accident, or tingling in your toes, or even digestive problems at the moment but the damage has been done. That injury has been delivered, that trauma has been felt by the body and the damage will continue to worsen until it's addressed. Just like going to the dentist and only after an x-ray they alert you to the fact that you have a cavity despite the fact that you don't feel pain, not having symptoms does not mean a person is healthy.

We are under a lot of stress in this country: emotionally, financially and physically. Every person on the planet is physically under the effects of gravity. It all takes a toll on the body from the type of work we do, to the long days of sitting and the emotional stress of deadlines. An unhealthy diet also puts stress on our body decreasing the nutrition required for us to repair and function properly. So, when you fall, are involved in a car accident or sports injury this compounds all the other stressors. When the body experiences constant stress we adapt, and our body begins to figure out new ways to handle the ongoing demands we place on it. This compensation further reduces the normal operations the body performs to keep us alive. The injury can be the last straw for your body and despite how you initially feel, the damage will be revealed over time. Therefore, following any type of trauma, you should get an evaluation just like you would for your car after an accident.

We're seeing younger kids with serious injuries to their spine caused by sports, slips or falls and especially heavy backpacks. Sports are great for kids to participate in, but they can also cause trauma to their bodies. Injuries accumulate over time. Regardless of whether they injure their knee, head or spine, because they're young they might not feel the injuries and damage to their body gets worse and worse over time as they get older. It's important to have the right equipment and protection for the body because we only get one of those. In order to prevent or have faster healing following an injury coaches can provide proper conditioning and a thorough understanding of the mechanics of how to play the game (how to take a hit versus being hit).

It's important that younger kids be taught what the spine and the nervous system do in the body. If they understood that any slips, falls or sports injuries could result in damage to their body later and that they should alert someone of these injuries when they occur, this could minimize any long-term damage. We get oil changed every three to five thousand miles, but we are trained to only go to the doctor when we're sick. Our goal would be to revolutionize this and help people understand more about their body and have less tolerance for these nagging, annoying problems that they go through life experiencing.

Care for an athlete's body is no different; it is important to ensure the traumas faced don't accumulate and lead to something bigger when they're 30. For example, football players that see chiropractors, incorporate natural health care, and engage in extra conditioning often have greater longevity. They understand that they may get a knee injury but know it's going to heal faster because their body in general is working better. They don't have the accumulation of built up traumas which would slow down their healing.

We've worked as athletic trainers in high school and seen so many student athletes running on state-of-the-art tracks with the best material and shock absorption but regardless of this, many of them presented with improper body mechanics. For instance, we observed someone running knock kneed. Their whole foot leaning in so much that we wondered how they were walking, let alone running without pain. It's really important for coaches to understand the need for good body mechanics. They may want to bring in a physician that will volunteer their time and do a screening on these kids and say, ' Listen, Suzy's foot is turned in and that's going to actually cause problems on the knee and that's going to lead to hip problems and ultimately back problems. But we can do this one simple fairly inexpensive thing to correct that.'" Now that coach will get better performance out of her as an athlete and she'll have a better quality of life and more longevity in the sport.

So, sports injuries can make or break a person. Athletes can either be well-conditioned and see the right people to help them bounce back faster or they end up so de-conditioned. Rudy in the movie "Rudy" just kept taking all the hits but if a person in that position didn't have a healthy body then they wouldn't be able to get back up.

We feel it goes back to education and that's why we go out in the community so much and that's why we've written this book. We want to help people understand how the body is supposed to work. Our goal is to encourage people to start looking at their body symptoms in more depth and asking, "Is this normal? What I'm feeling – is this normal or I should I get this checked out?" They need to know that any trauma to the body ultimately has a consequence, so regardless of any current symptoms of pain they should be evaluated following any injury. Even if you have no symptoms damage has resulted and you have two choices: deal with it now or deal with it later.

Chapter 6

Neck Pain, Carpal Tunnel Syndrome And Migraines

In this chapter we want to share how important the nervous system is starting with the neck. Every single nerve in your body starts at the base of the brain and goes through the neck. The nerves in the neck go down in the shoulders, arms and hands. If the neck has a normal position it should be in to allow for adequate space for the spinal cord to sit in. If the curve isn't properly positioned, the person will experience problems. The spinal cord wouldn't have enough space to pass through there and the nerves wouldn't have adequate room to exit between every pair of bones like they're supposed to, it can negatively affect the function of those nerves.

Neck Pain

We all know somebody who is a "pain in the neck" and we've all woken up with a pain in the neck. In either case, we want to get rid of the situation. The neck is the head of the body; the brain is in the skull and the skull sits right on top of the neck. Coming off the brain is the spinal cord. The spinal cord and the brain have certain reflexes built-in that will keep your eyes level with the horizon so you can see where you are going.

Injuries and traumas can occur to the neck. For example, just being born can cause misalignment. Many children suffer from ear infections when they're young because of the birthing process. Hopefully a child will come out headfirst, but the doctor may have to twist and turn the baby's head to get their shoulders out. This often times causes the child's first bone to be misaligned and the nerves that come out of those bones control the drainage of the ears. This undetected nerve damage or pressure that is building up prevent the ears from draining properly and over time bacteria settles in there. They get antibiotics that may eliminate the "infection", but it does not eliminate the reason why the child has it.

Neck pain is a very common problem affecting up to 70% of the adult population at some point in life. Though there are specific causes of neck pain such as arising from a sports injury, a car accident or "sleeping crooked," the vast majority of the time, no direct cause can be identified and thus the term nonspecific is applied. There are many symptoms associated with patients complaining of neck pain and many of these symptoms can be confused with other conditions. Wouldn't it be nice to know what neck related symptoms are most likely to respond to chiropractic manipulation before the treatment has started? This issue has been investigated with very favorable results!

The ability to predict a favorable response to treatment has been termed, "clinical prediction rules" which in general, are usually made up of combinations of things the patient says and findings from exams. In a large study, data from about 20,000 patients receiving about 29,000 treatments, was collected and analyzed to find out what complaints responded well to chiropractic treatment. The results showed that the presence of any 4 of these 7 presenting complaints predicted an immediate improvement in 70-95% of the patients: 1. Neck pain; 2. Shoulder, arm pain; 3. Reduced neck, shoulder, arm movement; 4. Stiffness; 5. Headache; 6. Upper, mid back pain, and 7. None or one presenting symptom. Items not associated with a favorable immediate response included "numbness, tingling upper limbs," and "fainting, dizziness and light-headedness in 4-12% of the patients. The "take-home" message here is that was far more common to see a favorable response (70-95%) of the patients compared to an unfavorable response (4-12%), supporting the observation that most patients with neck complaints will respond favorably to chiropractic treatment.

So, what do we do as chiropractors when a patient presents with neck pain? First, after gathering preliminary information such as name, address and insurance information, a history of the presenting complaint is taken. This consists of information including what started the neck complaint (if you know), when it started, what makes it worse, what makes it better, the quality of pain (aches, stiff, numb, etc.), the location and if there is radiating complaints, the severity (0-10 pain scale), timing (such as worse in the morning, evening, etc.), and if there have been prior episodes. Various questionnaires are included that are scored so improvement down the road can be tracked and a past history that includes a medication list, past injuries or illnesses, family history and a systems review are standard. The exam includes vital signs (BP, pulse, height, weight, temperature and respiration), palpation, range of motion, orthopedic and neurological examination. X-ray and/or other "special tests" may also be included, when needed. A review of all the findings are discussed and after permission to treat is granted, a chiropractic adjustment may then be rendered. A list treatment options may include:

1. Adjustments;
2. Soft tissue therapy (trigger point stimulation, myofascial release);
3. Physical therapy modalities;
4. Posture correction exercises and other exercises/home self-administered therapies;
5. Education about job modifications;

6. Co-management with other health care providers if/when needed.

What exercises can you do for your neck?

Exercise for the neck is very important since weak muscles are related to many painful conditions of the neck and, can contribute to fatigue, irritability, headache, sleep loss, and more. When done correctly (perform slowly, staying within "reasonable" pain boundaries), they can increase your range of motion, reduce stiffness/tightness, and strengthen your neck muscles.

The exercises below combine range of motion (ROM) against light/partial resistance in 4 directions (forwards, backwards, and L/R side bending). To do these correctly: Similar to an arm-wrestling contest: 1. Push your head into your hand while moving the head to the end of the range, "…letting the head win" (See A, C, E, G). 2. Repeat this going back in the opposite direction by "letting the hand win" (see B, D, F, H), again, moving through the entire range of motion. ALWAYS push the head into the hands, Make sure you move the head against resistance in BOTH directions, 3 times each (A-B then B-A x3; C-D then D-C x3) then, (E-F then F-E x3, and lastly, G-H then H-G, x3 reps). The trick is doing this VERY slowly (to build motor control and coordination) and to move through the entire "comfortable" range of motion. Repeat 3x slowly. If pain worsens, lighten up on the amount of pressure used or, stop the movement just prior to the sharp pain onset. If you can't make it to the end of the movement due to pain, make a note of how many reps it took before the onset or increase of pain and how far you could move your head. Do 3 slow reps and then move to the next exercise direction.

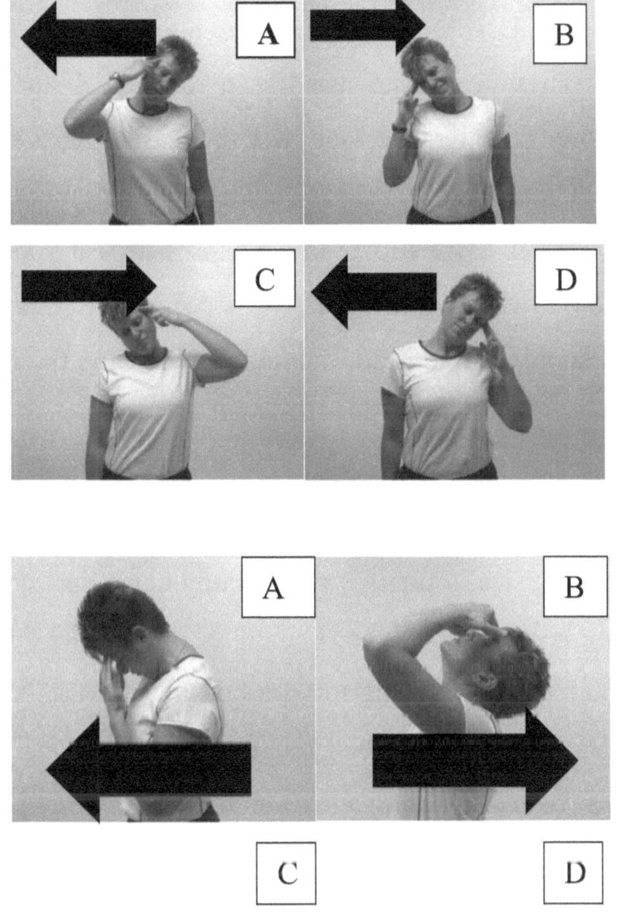

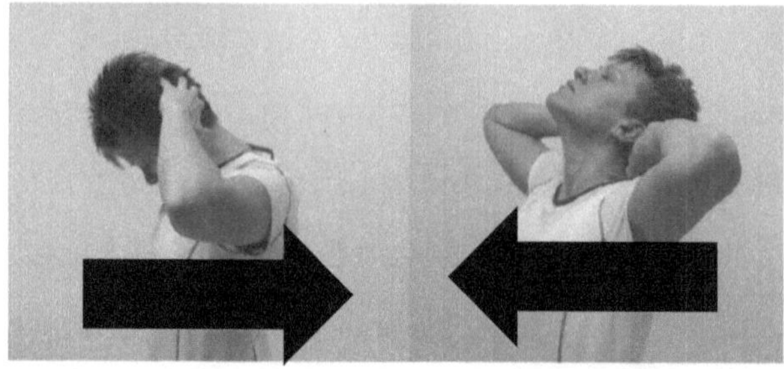

(The arrow represents the direction the head is moving, and the hands are resisting, but not stopping, the movement; Use light pressure through the full ROM)

These exercises can be performed 1 to 3x/day, according to tolerance, and will increase ROM, increase strength, and build coordination, all at the same time.

When there is pain in a person's neck it's important to find out what's causing it. The nerves in the neck control blood supply to the head, drainage of the ears, the function of your eyes, your ability to smell, the drainage of your sinuses and the movement of your neck muscles. Many patients come to us unable to turn their neck. They tell us, "I have to physically turn my whole body in my seat when I'm driving because I can't see behind me." Don't let that be an acceptable way of living for you because it doesn't have to be. It's a sign just like when your oil light comes on. It's your body's way of signaling a malfunction.

Carpal Tunnel

The nerves in the neck travel down into the arms and hands controlling blood flow, movement and sensation. If a person has a problem with their neck, the pressure on the nerves in the neck can cause problems in the hands. These nerve problems can cause a condition called Raynaud's which is a lack of normal circulation in the hands resulting in your hands turning red, white or blue depending on the body's reaction to cold or heat. More commonly, it can also lead to Carpal Tunnel Syndrome.

Most people's perception is that carpal tunnel is a repetitive-use injury, like in someone who's typing all day or a drummer or even a cashier who's constantly scanning items all day. While it's true those actions cause a lot of movement in the wrist it is attached to the shoulders, arms and hands (which all attach to the neck via the muscles). The nerves that go down into the wrist where that repetitive use is coming from start in the neck. If the joints in the wrist are not moving properly, that change in wrist mechanics is going to put more stress on certain parts of the wrist, certain nerves and blood vessels resulting in a compromised blood supply to that area resulting in carpal tunnel. So, if a person has had an injury or trauma to their neck that could pre-dispose them to carpal tunnel and they would develop symptoms much more rapidly. Someone who doesn't have a neck problem might not develop carpal tunnel despite having a repetitive motion type job.

In order to address wrist problems, some people will use a brace to keep the wrist straight so it's not moving. This can be temporarily helpful because it mechanically opens up the carpal tunnel that the nerves, arteries and veins go through. A splint is not going to fix the cause of the problem if it is due to an irritation to the nerves in the neck. While many doctors will say, "You have to stop drumming." or "You'll have to stop working on a computer." early in our careers we made it a goal to never tell somebody "You can't do this." We work to address the cause of your problem, so you don't have to stop doing the activities you love but learn how to perform them in a healthier way.

When struggling with carpal tunnel problems, doing surgery or just taking a medication like an anti-inflammatory is not going to fix the cause of the problem either. There is a big misconception that Carpal Tunnel is just caused by a circulatory problem. Circulation problems result in an alteration of temperature in the affected area. While this is often a factor in Carpal Tunnel, it's predominately a nerve problem.

When Dr. Howe was an intern; she went to a hospital for training. Someone walked up to the orthopedic surgeon we were with and said, "Doc, I have pain in my wrist." The surgeon replied, "Probably carpal tunnel we need you to schedule you for surgery." The whole class gasped! We began asking, "What about this orthopedic test? What about that test? What about blood supply? What about this?" And the doctor from our school just smiled and said, "That's the difference between what we do and what a surgeon does."

There's a time and place for every type of doctor. There are so many people that come to us thinking they're going to need surgery, but it ends up that surgery is not the most appropriate course of treatment for them. At the same time if someone does require surgery, we refer them to orthopedic surgeons or neurologists. We also encourage those patients to come back and really fix the cause of their problem once they've recovered from surgery.

Often individuals will have carpal tunnel surgery on their wrist because this is the area in which they feel the symptoms but that's not really the source of the problem. Even after surgery a person may still continue to have carpal tunnel symptoms because of the involvement of the nerves involved in the neck. We have many patients that we meet out in the community that say, "I've already had a surgery and I haven't gotten any better." And then we come to find out their neck is involved in the problem. Some patients have been diagnosed with double crush syndrome. Double crush syndrome is when the nerves are irritated in both the neck and the wrist. So just doing surgery at the wrist will not eliminate the cause of the problems.

So what can you do for carpal tunnel?

Carpal tunnel syndrome or, CTS, is a common condition that drives many patients to chiropractic clinics asking, "…what can chiropractic do for CTS?" As an overview, the following is a list of what you might expect when you visit a Doctor of Chiropractic for a condition like CTS:

1. **<u>A thorough history</u>** is VITALLY important as your doctor can ask about job related stressors, hobby related causes (such as carpentry or playing musical instruments), telephone work, or factory work – especially if it's fast and repetitive. Your doctor will also need to learn about your "co-morbidities" or, other conditions that can directly or indirectly cause CTS such as diabetes, thyroid disease, certain types of arthritis, certain medication side effects, and others.

2. **A Physical Exam** to determine the area(s) of nerve compression degree of severity. This may include ordering special tests such as EMG/NCV, if necessary.

3. **Treatment** can include manipulation, soft tissue release, PT modalities (e.g., electric stim., ultrasound).

4. **Home Therapies** are the main topic for this Health Update.

What can YOU do for CTS?

Here are some of the things that you, the CTS sufferer can self-manage:

1. **A Carpal tunnel splint** is primarily worn at night, keeping your wrist in a neutral or straight position. This position places the least amount of stretch on the nerves and muscle tendons that travel through the carpal tunnel at the wrist.

2. **Exercises** (Dose: 5-10 second holds, 5-10 repetitions, multiple times / day) such as:

   a. **The "Bear claw"** (keep the big knuckles of the hand straight but bend the 2 smaller joints of the fingers and thumb and alternate with opening wide the hand)

b. **Tight Fist / open hand** (fully open – spread and extend the fingers and then make a fist, with the hand).

c. **The upside-down palm** on wall wrist and forearm stretch (stand facing a wall; with the elbow straight, place the palm of your hand on the wall, fingers pointing down towards the floor. Try to bend the wrist to 90 degrees keeping the palm flat on the wall. Feel the stretch in the forearm – hold for 5-10 seconds. Reach across with the other hand and gently pull back on the thumb for an added stretch!

d. **Wrist range of motion**

(dorsiflexion/palmar flexion) – Place forearm on a table with wrist off the edge, palm down. Bend hand downward as far as possible, then upward. Repeat 5 or 10 times.

e. **Wrist range of motion**

(pronation/supination) – Place forearm and whole hand on table-- elbow bent 90°, palm flat on tabletop. Rotate the wrist and forearm so the back of hand is now flat on tabletop. Repeat 5 or 10 times.

f. **Neck Stretch.** Sit or stand with head facing forward. Side bend as far to the right as possible (approximate the right ear to right shoulder) and hold for 5 seconds. Reach over with the right hand to the left side of the head and gently pull further to the right to increase the stretch. Reverse instructions for the other side. Repeat 3 to 5 times. Consider other neck exercises if needed.

g. **Shoulder shrug and rotation.** Stand with arms at the sides. Shrug the shoulders up toward the ears, then squeeze the shoulder blades back, then downwards and then roll them forward. Do the whole rotation slowly and reverse the direction. Repeat 3 to 5 times. If you cannot comfortably do the whole rotation, just shrug the shoulders up and down.

h. **Pectoral stretch.** Stand in a doorway (or a corner of a room). Rest your forearms, including your elbows, on the doorframe, keeping your shoulders at a 90-degree angle. Lean forward until a stretch is felt in the chest muscles. Do not arch your back. Hold 20 seconds; repeat 5 times.

<u>Job modifications</u> are also VERY important but unfortunately, a topic for another time! In short, rotate job tasks (if possible), take mini-breaks, and use tools with handles that fit easily into the hands. Have a job station analysis completed if the above are not enough.

There are many non-surgical approaches to the treatment of CTS that should be utilized before surgery is considered, according to the American Academy of Neurology. In one study, 40% of neurologist polled recommended non-surgical care due to the potential side effects of surgery, some of which being severe, resulting in lengthy work loss post-surgically. A partial list of non-surgical care options includes:

1. Rest – Giving the inflamed CTS time to heal is therapeutic but not always an option.

2. Activity/job modifications – Avoiding certain activities or modifying them by taking breaks during the work day, slowing down the pace of the job, altering the position of the job task, such as propping up a part so that the wrists do not have to bend to the extremes, or when necessary, complete avoidance of the job task.

3.   Wrist Splint – This is a brace that maintains the wrist in a neutral position so it cannot easily bend. When the wrist flexes or extends, the pressure inside the carpal tunnel (on the palm side of the wrist) increases significantly, placing additional pressure on the already pinched median nerve. Wrist splints are especially useful at night.

4.   Nerve Gliding Exercises – These are exercises that stretch the wrist joint and muscle tendons (as well as the median nerve inside the carpal tunnel), with the objective of breaking adhesions that limit the normal glide or movement of the nerve in the forearm and wrist.

5.   Manual therapy techniques – These include manipulation of the arm including the forearm, wrist, and hand and sometimes the neck and shoulder, when needed. The objective is to improve the range of motion of the joints and soft tissues that may be participating in the process of median nerve pinching.

6.   Anti-inflammatory medication / nutrients – Medications include aspirin, ibuprofen, naproxen and similar prescription drugs. Nutritional options including herbs (such as ginger, turmeric, boswellia), digestive enzymes, and Vitamin B6 may also help. Ice is also anti-inflammatory and direct, on-the-skin ice massage is quite effective.

Carpal Tunnel Syndrome – Chiropractic vs. Medical Treatment

There are many patients who suffer from Carpal Tunnel Syndrome (CTS). In fact, CTS is one of the most common work-related injuries. In spite of multiple studies that show the benefits of chiropractic treatment with patients suffering from CTS, many medical doctors are unaware of the studies and still tell their patients that chiropractic treatment is either ineffective or may actually harm them. This unsupported ill advice can easily result in the patient not even considering chiropractic care as a potential effective form of treatment. This can be especially damaging to a patient who cannot tolerate anti-inflammatory medications such as Ibuprofen, Aleve, or aspirin. In fact, side effects secondary to stomach pain (gastritis and/or ulcer) can be quite common, especially at the recommended dose of 2400 mg / day. Moreover, if poor tolerance to these medications exists and an unsatisfying response to conservative medical treatment occurs, the "next step" offered to the patient may be surgery. Surgery that may have been avoidable had chiropractic treatment been considered on an equal par to non-surgical medical care.

There are several studies available that will enlighten those who simply are not aware of the effectiveness of chiropractic care in the treatment of CTS. In 1998, a 91 patient group was divided in half and treated for 9 weeks by either a non-surgical medical approach or by a chiropractic treatment approach. The medical approach included the use of 800 mg of Ibuprofen, 3x/day for 1 week, 2x/day for 1 week, and 800mg as needed to a maximum of 2400 mg/day dose for 7 weeks, as well as the use of a nighttime wrist splint. The chiropractic group utilized manipulation of the bony joints and soft tissues of the spine and upper extremity for 3x/week for 2 weeks, 2x/week for 3 weeks, and 1x/week for 4 weeks, in addition to ultrasound over the carpal tunnel and a wrist splint at night. It was reported that BOTH the medical and the chiropractic patient groups did equally well stating, "significant improvement in perceived comfort and function, nerve conduction and finger sensation."

In 2007, two different chiropractic approaches were compared and found to both be equally effective in improving nerve conduction, wrist strength, and wrist motion as well as patient satisfaction and daily activity function. These improvements were maintained for 3 months in both groups equally as well. Another study reported significant improvements in strength, range of motion, and pain after chiropractic treatment was given to 25 patients diagnosed with CTS. The majority of the patients reported continued improvements for 6 months or more. There are other studies, but I think the point is obvious – chiropractic treatment helps patients with CTS.

The type of treatment that one may receive when being treated by a chiropractor includes manipulation of the bony joints of the neck and upper extremity. The objective of this is to improve the mobility of the joints and loosen the muscles through which the nerves pass, particularly, the median nerve that runs through the carpal tunnel and innervates the 2nd to 4th fingers. There are several exercises of both stretching and strengthening types that strive for similar goals. Physical therapy modalities such as low-level laser therapy have reported beneficial results.   Other modalities such as ultrasound, interferential current (IFC), ice massage/cupping over the tunnel, and others may also be utilized. Nighttime wrist splints or braces also help to keep the wrist straight so that prolonged bending of the wrist at night is not possible.   There may be other treatment approaches that your chiropractic physician may suggest on an individual case basis.

A recent study in the Journal of Manipulative and Physiological Therapeutics compared two different conservative treatments for patients with mild to moderate carpal tunnel symptoms. One treatment was the Graston technique, which uses an instrument to rub the forearm, wrist and hand areas to breakdown scar tissue and adhesions. In the other treatment a chiropractor applied deep pressure by hand to the same areas. These treatments are thought to release tight muscles and myofascial restrictions.

The patients got the treatments twice each week for four weeks followed by one treatment a week for two additional weeks. The patients also did at-home stretching exercises. They did not use common conservative treatments such as wrist splints and anti-inflammatory medications.

After both interventions, there were objective improvements to nerve conduction latencies (nerve function), wrist strength, and wrist motion. The patient symptoms of pain also improved, and both groups reported high satisfaction with the care they received.

Despite surgery being in widespread use in the US for carpal tunnel syndrome, it is important for conservative treatments to be tried prior to an invasive operation.

The surgical complication rates are low but when they do occur, can be devastating. In addition to direct surgery costs, one has to also consider disability payments (not working), and rehabilitation that may take several weeks. These costs can be substantial. For this reason, many medical doctors recommend conservative treatments first.

Of all the conservative options, manual therapy by a chiropractor is an excellent choice. It comes without the side effects associated with long-term use of medications.

Headaches

We have a lot of patients that come to see us because they have unresolved headaches. The nerves in the neck control blood supply to the brain. People realize that most headaches are due to blood flow problems, but they think the blood vessels are like a straw and the blood just flows through it. What people don't realize is that the blood vessels have muscles in them. The muscles in the blood vessels rely on the nerves from the neck to control and contract them in order to squeeze the blood and open up so that the blood can move through. A person with an injury to their neck, like from the birthing process, experiencing a slip or a fall, or a car accident, may have pressure on those nerves and that could be contributing to the headaches they are experiencing.

We had a 22-year-old gymnast come into our wellness center. Gymnasts are constantly learning new things and no matter how good they are, they fall. Dr. Howe has worked on an Olympic gymnast who knew that she needed to see a chiropractor before she went to the Olympics. This person knew that they should get care and that's what allowed them to have longevity in a sport that can really beat you up your body. This young gymnast also had headaches every single day for weeks prior to being seen. Doctors had resorted to heavy duty medication. They were putting her on birth control pills and all different kinds of things to try to change her hormones and control the pain. As soon as Dr. Howe looked at her she could see the girl didn't have normal posture in her neck and it wasn't because she wasn't sitting up straight. It was the way her muscles were holding her to compensate for something that was happening higher up in her neck. A simple x-ray showed she sustained an injury to her neck. We were able to help get her on the road to feeling well. But this poor girl has been suffering for 21 days with a headache hoping it was going to get better. Thinking she could tough it out. In reality, there was a problem that would have gotten worse had her aunt not sent her into the clinic.

Migraines

Migraines can be so debilitating. We've helped a lot of people with migraines. It's one of our favorite things to help people with because they are so crippling. Unfortunately, those suffering with migraines get to a level where they are told they are "as good as they're going to be". It is not unusual to hear sufferers say, "I don't get them as often" or "They are not as intense" or "I don't black out" or "I don't miss work" – that becomes people's new norm, their new level of acceptability. When we can help them see, they don't have to live like that and understand the reason they are suffering, they tear up. We can often show them in black and white on an x-ray why they're having this problem. It's great to be on that journey with them. Many times, patients come in and they're crabby or down on themselves. We tell our staff, "Just wait until they start to feel better, you'll see their real personality come out."

Dr. Howe's sister sprained her ankle one time. It was when our office was being built so we didn't have an x-ray machine. So, she took her to the hospital in the middle of the night. In the waiting room with us was a person who had been there for five hours dealing with a migraine. And this wasn't the first time. Each time they tried to treat their migraines with more and more medications, but they weren't getting any relief.

There was a previous study were doctors who had to blacklist patients from headache medication because they were having what's called 'bounce-back headaches'. These patients were taking so much medication, it was changing the physiology in their body. Their chemical makeup was actually creating more headaches. All medications have side effects and are processed through the liver. The liver has other jobs to perform as well, so for it to have to be filtering all these medications is not healthy. Pretty soon the body does develop a tolerance.

At our centers, instead of adding more medications to patients, we work to find the cause of the problem. We had a woman that came in who was in her 50s. She had been suffering from headaches for the last 10 years. Her headaches would last two or three days. She would be fine for a day or two and then the headache would come back again. She told us that she had been to a chiropractor without success and didn't want traditional chiropractic care. We understood what she meant. Why do the same thing and think something different is going to happen? We asked her if anyone had ever looked at what she was eating. Her reply was, "No. Why would it matter what I'm eating because I get them no matter what I eat." We performed a workup on her and found out that she had a sensitivity to corn. When she was newly retired, she and her husband were eating out a lot more where there are processed foods and you don't necessarily know what's in it. The foods at restaurants aren't always like what someone would cook at home. Armed with this new information we took her off of corn and corn-based products and put her on a detox program.

In the first three days, she noticed that she didn't have the headaches anymore. And it got better and from there. She understood more about how she could prevent them. We also worked with her spine and nervous system to make sure that her body didn't have the old physical stresses that it had before.

Her husband came in one day. He was a big, intimidating, gruff kind of guy and he said, "I need to talk to you." His wife didn't have an appointment. He just showed up unannounced and we thought, "All right. Let's see what's going on." He came in the room and he started crying and he said, "I have to thank you so much for giving my wife back to me." We asked him what he meant. He replied, "She's the sweetest lady and then she was dealing with these headaches. We didn't go out and do things and I could see she was miserable, and I didn't know how to help her. It made me feel like I'm less of a man because I didn't know what to do for her. And it is my wife and I'm watching her suffer." Unfortunately, within the next couple of months he passed away. And she got those couple of months with him completely headache-free when no one else— not the Diamond Headache Clinic or Mayo Clinic could help her. She'd been on every kind of medication. She had learned meditation and biofeedback, and nothing had helped her and here it was literally something that was going into her mouth every day. They were both so grateful. It's such a rewarding opportunity to be part of changing and improving people's quality of life.

Migraines are so hard on the body emotionally and physically. Plus, the family of the patient has to watch them suffer, often for a long time. Most sufferers can get real relief and no longer have to live with headaches. There was only one person in our careers we have not been able to completely eliminate their headaches. This woman loaded jets for a living and constantly had that fuel toxifying her system. By changing up her diet and working on her spine and nervous system, she was able to control her headaches a lot more instead of having them all day every day. She actually loved her job; she just didn't like the headaches that came with them.

Migraines are usually characterized by unilateral, throbbing headaches aggravated by movement or straining. Typically, migraine pain is localized at a certain spot, but it sometimes varies from attack to attack and even within a single episode.

Migraines can cause:

nausea and vomiting

evoke visual disturbances,

numbness,

tingling and weakness of the limbs,

inability to speak properly, and cause

intolerance to light and noise.

Migraine attacks can begin at any age, but most often they appear between 20-30 years, and begin to calm down after 50.

You may be more likely to get migraines due to

heredity,

hormonal changes at puberty,

frequent stresses,

fatigue, and

intense mental activity, among other factors.

As you can see by the story above, chiropractic can be effective against migraines, when the Doctor performs a series of manipulations aimed at the spine to correct deviations that can cause migraines.

Dizziness/Vertigo

Dizziness is a sensation of lightheadedness, faintness or unsteadiness. Vertigo has a rotational, spinning component and is the perception of movement, either of the self or surrounding objects. Dizziness can be linked to a wide array of problems and is commonly linked to blood flow irregularities from cardiovascular problems. Other causes could include: vestibular problems (ear), nervous system disorders, medications and even osteoarthritis. Degeneration of the vertebrae in the neck can create pressure on both the nerves and blood vessels which can interfere with blood supply to the brain.

Dr. Schultz had a patient who began suffering with dizziness that produced such severe symptoms that she would suddenly vomit profusely causing her to pull off the road. The accompanying visual disturbances, spinning and tunnel vision incapacitated her to the point where she had to call for a ride home. Her main reason for seeking our care was big toe pain. Upon examination and x-rays, Dr. Schultz discovered that despite three other doctors inability to definitively find the cause of these symptoms, this patient had spinal cord stenosis (narrowing) due to previous spinal trauma. This problem resulted in pressure on the nerves and blood vessels supplying the head, neck and brain.

The spinal rehabilitation corrective program recommended by Dr. Schultz had such an impact on this patient that within the first two months the patient reported a significant reduction of the intensity and frequency of her episodes and after three months she was episode-free. A consultation with this patient eighteen months after starting care found her to have no recurrence of her symptoms.

Chapter 7

Mid-back Pain

Most people are familiar with lower back pain, they don't realize how much the mid-back is an integral part of the body. Attached to the mid-back are the shoulders, rib cage, and nerves that run through the thoracic spine. These nerves control many different essential body functions including breathing and the heart rate and metabolism; all crucial to staying alive.

The mid-back includes the shoulders and the arms connected to them. These are important for keeping a person upright and especially useful in keeping the head on the neck. The ribs are attached to the spine just like the joints of the fingers line up. There are muscles in between each set of ribs that help the rib cage expand when breathing in and relax when you breathe out. If one of those ribs suddenly becomes misaligned, those muscle spasms. This can produce a piercing or stabbing sensation from the back of the body to the front when a deep breath is taken. This stabbing pain can be mistaken for a heart attack or gallbladder problem (these must be ruled out).

If a patient were concerned about this kind of issue and sought treatment through a traditional medical doctor, anti-inflammatories, pain killers and muscle relaxants may be prescribed. These will take hours or days to work.

When seeking relief for this same issue from a Chiropractor, the Dr., who has also taken the Hippocratic Oath and practices "first, do no harm," would make sure it wasn't a heart attack or something more serious. Then the Dr. can find the rib that is misaligned, or the muscles involved and test them. If pushing on the rib or muscles reproduces the pain the misalignment is diagnosed, treated immediately; providing instantaneous relief in many cases.

The thoracic spine nerves are responsible for providing function to the heart, lungs and many organs that control our metabolism. It is essential to normal operation of our body that these nerves work properly. When the spine or ribs are misaligned and put pressure on these nerves we commonly see other symptoms in the body manifest. These might include things like asthma, acid reflux, or heart arrythmias.

Asthma

The Center For Disease Control (CDC) states that approximately 9 people per day die from asthma. The incidence and prevalence of asthma increased 15% in the last decade. One in eleven children and one in twelve adults has asthma according to the CDC's 2012 Asthma Control Program. Today's environment has many more pollutants and toxins than it has ever had. There are 84,000 pollutants in the air, food, and water we come into contact with every day. A child's immune system is not as strong as an adults. Therefore, certain foods and environmental exposures can cause a buildup of toxins and poisons when not properly digested and metabolized.

When an adult is exposed to toxins and poisons the body responds by surrounding the toxin with fat and water to protect itself from damage. Toxins are also processed throughout the liver and expelled from the body through breathing, sweating, urinating and bowel movements. Since children don't usually have excess body fat to store the toxins or a system experienced in handling them, they rely more the lungs (and liver) for excretion. This extra strain on the lungs can produce signs and symptoms of asthma.

Additionally, more and more kids today are using electronics (iPhones, iPads, tablets and computers) spending a significant amount of time in a hunched over posture instead of running and playing. This poor posture impacts the thoracic spine nerves. So, asthma in children can be caused in part by posture; part by chemicals; and certainly slips, falls, accidents, and things that create undetected nerve damage. Sometimes the asthma is the first sign that there's been an injury to the nervous system or the spine.

Protecting Children from Developing Asthma

While it may be difficult to protect children from slips and falls there are steps a parent can take to protect their kids and help prevent asthma. As previously shared, improving posture and limiting electronic game play can certainly help but it is even more important to understand how the body works. Some of the foods used to fuel the body can produce chemical stress. That's why it's so important to educate and train children at a young age to put good, wholesome foods into their body so it can work to the best of its potential. A race car driver wouldn't put sugar water in their gas tank. They would choose a high-functioning fuel for their car – and the same needs to be done for the body. It's always about striking a balance. If a parent is going to give their kids hotdogs they might also include broccoli. If their child desires chips they could try gluten-free pretzels with some humus which also provides some protein from garbanzo beans. The old adage, "you are what you eat" is so true and parents can help when they lead by example. If a child does have a slip or a fall it's important to bring them to see an expert to evaluate the function of the nervous system and the movement of the spine. They can ensure there's not something that needs to be addressed now rather than let the damage go undetected. This ensures your body maintains the ability to do its job.

Asthma is the most common chronic disease in childhood affecting over 7 million children (and about 24 million adults in the US). Asthma affects the airways causing them to tighten and fill with mucus.

Pathophysiology of asthma. Asthma occurs as a result of 3 main mechanisms. These include; bronchial hyperactivity or hyperresponsiveness, airway inflammation and airflow obstruction. Bronchial hyperactivity involves an excess response to numerous stimuli both endogenous and exogenous. The degree of hyperactivity's depend on the severity of the disease. Airway inflammation can be acute, subacute or chronic. This leads to a reduction in the size of the airways. Airway obstruction is contributed by increased mucus secretion into the airways, smooth muscle hyperplasia and the disquamation of the epithelium.

Signs and symptoms of asthma. Asthma symptoms can range from mild to severe. They include: -

Wheezing

Coughing

Shortness of breath

Chest tightness

Chest pains.

There are some non-specific symptoms that occur in infants and young children such as

persistent cough with colds,

recurrent pneumonia,

bronchitis

bronchiolitis,

and recurrent chest rattling.

Different patients have different severity and triggers for asthma. Some patients may have symptoms daily while others may only experience asthma with an infection like a cold or during intense exercise.

Early warning signs of asthma include;

coughing after exercise,

shortness of breath,

frequent cough (especially at night),

and feeling over-tired while exercising. Asthma classification. Asthma can be classified in 4 groups based on the severity of the symptoms. Intermittent asthma, mild asthma, moderate asthma, and severe persistent asthma.

Chiropractic treatment of asthma.

Chiropractic treatment of asthma involves manipulation of the spinal cord to correct misalignments and to relieve pressure on the nerves that innervate the respiratory organs. The pressure on the nerves leads to malfunction of the organs which may lead to the intrinsic form of asthma. Spinal manipulation has benefited asthma patients in terms of improving asthma symptoms, enhancing endocrine effects and even improving the patients immunologic capacity.

In one study it was noted that chiropractic treatment reduced patients' symptoms from 4 attacks a month to only 1 attack a month. This reduced the cost of medication by about 70%.

Chiropractic treatment also improved accompanying symptoms like depression and anxiety experienced by asthma patients. Chiropractic treatment also have positive biochemical and physiological changes that have a long-term effect on asthma management. Patients with juvenile onset asthma reported a significant improvement after just 5 chiropractic treatments over a period of 1 month. Patients with bronchial asthma reported an increased peak flow rate and vital capacity after the third chiropractic treatment.

Patients in 3 clinical trials have reported that they have experienced improved quality of life and lessening of symptoms of asthma after getting exposed to chiropractic care.

The frequency of their asthma attacks decreased, and there were fewer respiratory muscle spasms caused by asthma.

There has also been a decrease in the asthmatic attack episodes of the patients who have undergone chiropractic care.

Digestive Disorders

The nerves housed in the mid-back additionally control the digestive system. Thirteen out of the 26 pairs of nerves in the body, control the digestion and metabolism. Digestion is critical for every function in the body. Proper posture and movement of this area are essential to overall body health as the thoracic spine is the bridge between the neck and low back. Built-up stress in this area inhibits proper communication between the brain and the rest of the body. Spicy foods are often thought to be the culprit of many digestive disorders, but that isn't necessarily the case. Foods like coffee, pop, tea, chocolate, citrus, and really spicy foods have a more acidic pH. Excess acid causes the body to release nutrients that are basic or alkaline. These nutrients help neutralize the acid preventing it from burning a hole through the stomach. Vitamins and minerals come from the foods we eat, and any supplements added to the diet. Properly digested foods provide nutrients for energy and healing of the body.

If you have a digestive problem and have ruled out spicy foods or infection as the culprit, you might have a problem with the nervous system in the mid-back. In order to digest even one bite of food, the brain must signal different digestive system organs and glands to release their enzymes to systematically breakdown the food into the vitamins and minerals our body needs in order to function. If the brain is unable to properly communicate with the digestive system this results in partially digested food floating around the body. This can trigger food sensitivities, gas and bloating – issues many mistakenly believe to be "age-related". These problems may actually have nothing to do with age but instead can be the result of injury and trauma to the nerves affecting the digestive system that hadn't been previously identified or addressed.

Preventing Mid-Back Pain

Stress and strain occur on the mid-back through poor posture, working, driving, carrying a heavy briefcase or luggage or wearing heavy backpacks. You may not even realize these activities can cause problems until something like a misaligned rib or a muscle spasm drops you to your knees.

Prevention of misalignment is best done by keeping motion in the thoracic spine. If the mid-back doesn't have motion, the neck and the lower back will never move or work properly. Problems in these areas cannot truly be eliminated until the mid-back motion and alignment are addressed. This is accomplished through our Spinal Rehabilitation program. If a person has problems with their mid-back, it's important to have it corrected because it's connected to so many other parts and functions of the body. A mid-back misalignment isn't always the cause of stabbing pain in the chest, asthma or digestive problems but when looking at the cause of these problems, it needs to be considered before thinking it is some horrible disorder or disease. It's important that problems in this area don't go undetected and at the same time relief may be closer than you think.

Chapter 8

Why Is Lower Back Pain So Common?

This question has plagued all of us, including researchers for a long time! Could it be because we're all inherently lazy and don't exercise enough? Or maybe it's because we have a job that's too demanding on our back? To properly address this question, here are some interesting facts:

1. The prevalence of low back pain (LBP) is common, as 70-85% of ALL PEOPLE have back pain that requires treatment of some sort at some time in life.
2. On a yearly basis, the annual prevalence of back pain averages 30% and once you have back pain, the likelihood of recurrence is high.
3. Back pain is the most common cause of activity limitation in people less than 45 years of age.
4. Back pain is the 2nd most frequent reason for physician visits, the 5th ranking reason for hospital admissions, and is the 3rd most common cause for surgical procedures.
5. About 2% of the US workforce receives compensation for back injuries annually.
6. Similar statistics exist for other countries, including the UK and Sweden.

Low back pain can cause anything from a generalized ache to a sharp stabbing pain to numbness, or weakness down the leg. All of these symptoms need to be evaluated in order to identify the root cause. Each problem is treated differently with medications or surgery based on whatever a doctor may recommend. Before treatment is prescribed it's important to identify the cause so the best solution can be found.

If weakness down the leg is experienced it is important to determine if this is caused from a problem with the lower back. Often symptoms experienced are just the tip of the iceberg, but they are the body's way of saying, "there's a problem here." The hidden cause of that problem is what needs to be discovered or else the symptoms are all that is being treated. Back pain symptoms could be treated with over the counter pain relievers, medication, a heating pad, ice, and many other ways. But if the true cause of the problem isn't addressed, the symptoms will continue, and a person will start to feel as though they have a back problem and alter their life rather than uncover the cause of it and treat the main cause.

Disc Problems

Lower back pain can often be connected to a herniated disc, spinal stenosis and even hormone problems (that's right). The entire spine is made of twenty-six moveable bones and in between each pair of bones is a disc that is a gel-like substance mostly made of water. The disc separates the two bones and between those bones a nerve exits on both the left and right side of the spine. The height of the disc dictates the size of the hole each nerve travels through from the spinal cord to the area of the body it is responsible for controlling. The structure of the spine is such that as the spinal column goes from top to bottom the size of both the discs and bones increases. Therefore, the bones and discs in the low back are the largest and this is important because this is where a person's center of gravity is located.

The joints of the human body are made to never wear out, however, because gravity is constantly pushing down on our body, if a person's body is not properly aligned then it will bear weight on the spinal joints unevenly and inappropriately resulting in break down. Irregular wear and tear on the joints result in premature breakdown of the discs this called Degenerative Disc Disease. When degenerative disc disease, arthritis, or any other number of degenerative problems occur, it is often because warning signs like pain, tingling and numbness have been ignored. Following an injury, the body manifests symptoms as a result of the trauma it experienced. For instance, when you roll your ankle (which results in a stretch, tear or pull of a ligament) the result is swelling. The purpose of the swelling is to limit motion of the injured area as well as supply it with new blood to promote healing. When spinal joints are misaligned from slips, falls or injuries of any kind, they too display signs of the damage. These signs may include: leaning to one side (antalgic posture), pain, limping, referred pain down the leg (sciatica), digestive problems (because of pressure on a nerve that contributes to the digestive system) or even lack of pain (due to numbness) or the person may choose to ignore these symptoms and "push" through them.

Ignoring symptoms can cause more damage than one might think. It's like driving with your check engine light on and ignoring it, sooner or later your car will breakdown. The same is true of your body, these symptoms indicate something bigger is happening. When a person has heart problems, they receive warning signs and symptoms. They may experience discomfort in their chest, get indigestion or feel lightheaded. As a society we have been educated about these warning signs and know they can indicate heart problems that need to be addressed immediately.

Our society is lacking in education on the long-term ramifications of untreated low back pain. The goal of our wellness center is to change this through patient education. We train our patients to prevent this suffering and to recognize the warning signs and symptoms. They can avoid experiencing excruciating pain; shooting pain down the leg and difficulty sitting or lying without severe pain. These can all be prevented when the root problem of low back pain is identified and treated.

The Differences Between Slipped and Herniated Discs

Mayo clinic refers to a herniated disc (sometimes called a "slipped disc") as a problem with one of the rubbery cushions (discs) between the individual bones (vertebrae) that stacks up to make your spine. Think of a disc like the jelly filling in a donut. When you push on one side of the donut the jelly is going to squirt out of the other side. Gravity itself pushes straight down on the spine and discs. If the joints of the spine aren't lined up properly, they can become jammed and move improperly. If bones in the spine are misaligned, they put pressure on one side or part of the disc. It would be similar to driving down the road with tires that are not aligned properly. This would cause rubbing, pulling or a shimmying in a car. The same thing happens in the body. The misalignment and pressure on the disc can feel like a pinching or a shooting pain; a dull ache; constant pain or pain with movement.

A herniated disc is also referred to as ruptured disc or a slipped disc. This disorder may cause great pain, and in some cases, may lead to permanent nerve damage if not treated. To understand about this condition, you must first know how the backbone works, of which the disc is a part.

The backbone stretches from the bottom of the skull towards the base of the pelvis known as the sacrum. It is comprised of 33 individual hard bone components which are called vertebrae. The vertebrae are held together by tendons, ligaments, and muscle. The vertebrae are interconnected in such a way that it makes the backbone flexible, which enables us to jump, bend, stretch, twist, and flip.

The difference between slipped and herniated discs differ in size according to their location in the spine. For example, the discs within the lower spine, are bigger compared to the ones in the neck region. These discs are categorized according to the location where they are The discs in the neck region are known as cervical discs. The discs within the upper back region are called thoracic discs. The discs within the lower back region are called lumbar discs. Typically, the discs are a perfect fit within the vertebrae and so are in proper alignment.

These discs are full of fluid which enable the discs to act as shock supports that soften the impact of stresses the backbone is subjected to. As part of aging, the fluid inside the disc stiffens, making the disc much less flexible. The disc gradually becomes very hard and unyielding, making them vulnerable to injury.

When a disc is herniated, the middle area of the disc enlarges, exerting pressure on the delicate spinal nerves in the spinal cord.

What are the symptoms of disc problems? They usually vary considerably depending on its location as well as the severity. Majority of people who have been diagnosed with damaged discs do not portray any symptoms. This can be interpreted to mean that there are no signs and symptoms at all. Nevertheless, in general, some of the signs to watch out for include: back pain, pain that radiates down your legs, extreme pain associated with sitting down or bending over for a long period, extreme pain associated with activities such as sneezing or coughing, and pins and needles in the legs or arms or even numbness.

Is My Disc Slipped or Herniated?

When your disc is slipped, the inner jelly-like nucleus is pushed out of place, but it is still contained within the walls of the disc. This typically causes back pain and may cause sciatica, which is pain or numbness and tingling in your leg.

A herniated disc is considered a more serious condition, and results when the inner nucleus of the disc is pushed so far out of place that it exits the annulus surrounding the disc. The inner disc material is then free to press up against spinal nerves.

If your MRI indicates that you have a slipped or herniated disc, you should have a thorough musculoskeletal examination by a licensed chiropractor who is trained to assess your condition. Your chiropractor can then prescribe the correct treatments to help you decrease your back pain and get you back to your previous level of activity and function.

Spinal Stenosis

Stenosis means narrowing that occurs almost anywhere in the body. Spinal stenosis refers to a narrowing of the spinal canal (where the spinal cord runs through the spine) or the holes the spinal nerves exit through (foramina).

There are two types of spinal stenosis: functional and structural stenosis. Structural stenosis is where bone grows in the canal that the spinal cord sits in or on the foramina. The only chance at possibly repairing that requires surgery. The most common cause of functional stenosis can be seen on an x-ray taken in a seated position. A seated x-ray shows the body in its weakest position. A patient is less likely to try to suck in their stomach, tuck in their rear end or throw back their shoulders when they are seated. When we look at these x-rays, we see bones that have shifted in an inappropriate fashion. This results in a functional stenosis; meaning that because the bones have shifted, the canal appears smaller, the spinal cord is now being squeezed and that can ultimately create very serious symptoms. Through treatment we can often restore normal alignment to the bones resulting in a more optimal size of the canal.

Our goal is to identify the cause of the stenosis, whether it is structural or functional. Many patients experience great results with our therapy and significantly reduce their symptoms without surgical intervention.

We address the spine as a whole. When a person has a problem with their low back, many times during a physical examination and through x-rays we see there's an underlying problem in their neck as well. If we only evaluated where the pain was, we may miss the cause of the problem. Our spinal rehab therapy is delivered to the entire spine because the entire spine is connected

Hormones

The general public is unaware that the nerves in the lower spine control not only the muscles of the low back and legs, but also the function of the bladder, kidneys and reproductive system. Many women come to our clinic with hot flashes, PMS or severe cramping during their menstrual cycle. When we ask them about these symptoms they say, " well, I'm 40 (or I'm 50) or I would expect my libido to be compromised because I'm stressed and fatigued or everyone in my family has really painful periods." Many men come to our office with low testosterone, waking up a lot at night to go to the bathroom, or erectile dysfunction. When we examine them, we often discover that they don't have a normal curve in their low back, which means the bones are shifted and have compromised function of their nerves. This problem with the nerves can have a tremendous effect on hormone balance, contribute to incontinence and decreased libido.

Our clinic specializes in evaluating hormone levels and working with a compounding pharmacy that can make personalized medications based on their exam findings.

This method ensures that each patient receives the balance of the specific hormone(s) their body requires vs. something "most women or men" respond favorably to.

By evaluating the spine in addition to hormone levels, we can often work with a patient's other doctor or make other recommendations for them in addition to what their doctor has recommended. This can provide the balance they truly need and help them regain the function of their body.

What can you do about it?

Here are some very practical exercises to do, "…for the rest of our lives." Start with the easy ones!

1. Easy (Level 1): **<u>Standing eyes open/closed</u>** - Start with the feet shoulder width apart, look straight ahead to get your balance and then close the eyes and try not to sway counting to 30 by, "…one thousand one, one thousand two, one thousand three, etc." Repeat this with your feet closer together until they touch each other. You can make this harder by standing on a pillow or cushion -- but don't start that way!

2. Medium (Level 2): **<u>Lunges</u>** - from a similar starting position as #1, step forwards with one leg and squat slightly before returning back to the start position. Repeat

this 5x with each foot/leg. As you progress, you can take a longer stride and/or squat down further with each repetition. You can even hold onto light dumbbells and/or close your eyes to make it more challenging.

3. Hard (Level 3): **<u>Rocker or wobble board exercises</u>** - use a platform that rocks back & forth or, wobbles in multiple directions. Rock back and forth, eyes open and then closed, once you get comfortable on the board. You can rotate your body on the board, standing straight ahead (12 o'clock) followed by 45-degree angles as you work your way around in a circle at 45-degree increments (12, 1:30, 3, 4:30, 6, 7:30, 9, 10:30 and back to noon). Repeat these eyes open and closed. The Wii Balance board is a fun way to exercise – check that out as well.

You can "improvise" and mix up different exercises and create your own routine. Just remember, stay safe, work slowly until you build up your confidence and keep challenging yourself. Of course, you should do these first under the supervision of your chiropractor to make sure they are appropriate for your low back pain.

Does Chiropractic Work? - What Will My Insurance Company Say?

If chiropractic care helps patients get better faster and costs the patient and/or insurance company less, shouldn't EVERY low back pain patient FIRST see a chiropractor before any other type of doctor? That is in fact, what should be done, based on a recent report!

A recent report was delivered on the impact on population, health and total health care spending. It was found the addition of chiropractic care for the treatment of neck and low back pain "...will likely increase value-for-dollar in US employer-sponsored health benefit plans." Authored by an MD and an MD/PhD, and commissioned by the Foundation for Chiropractic Progress, the findings are clear; chiropractic care achieves higher satisfaction and superior outcomes for both neck and low back pain in a manner more cost effective than other commonly utilized approaches.

The study reviews the fact that low back and neck pain are extremely common conditions consuming large amounts of health care dollars. In 2002, 26% of surveyed US adults reported having back pain in the prior 3 months, 14% had neck pain and the lifetime prevalence of back pain was estimated at 85%. LBP accounts for 2% of all physician office visits where only routine examinations, hypertension, and diabetes result in more. Annual national spending is estimated at $85 billion in the US with an inflation-adjusted increase of 65% compared to 1997. Treatment options are diverse ranging from rest to surgery, including many various types of medications. Chiropractic care, including spinal manipulation and mobilization, is reportedly also widely utilized with almost half of all patients with persisting back pain seeking chiropractic treatment.

In review of the scientific literature, it is noted that 1) chiropractic care is at least as effective as other widely used therapies for low back pain; 2) Chiropractic care, when combined with other modalities such as exercise, appears to be more effective than other treatments for patients with neck pain. Other studies reviewed reported patients who had chiropractic coverage included in their insurance benefits found lower costs, reduced imaging studies, less hospitalizations, and surgical procedures compared to those with no chiropractic coverage. They then utilized a method to compare medical physician care, chiropractic physician care, physiotherapy-led exercise and, manipulation plus physiotherapy-led exercise for low back pain care. They found adding chiropractic physician care is associated with better outcomes at "…equivalent to an incremental cost-effectiveness ratio of $1837 per QALY (Quality-adjusted Life Year)."

When combined with exercise, chiropractic physician care was also found to be very cost-effective when compared to exercise alone. This combined approach would achieve improved health outcomes at a cost of $152 per patient, equivalent to an "incremental cost-effectiveness ratio of $4591 per QALY." When comparing the cost effectiveness of chiropractic care with or without exercise even at 5 times the cost of the care they utilized in their analysis, it was still found to be "substantially more cost-effective" compared to the other approaches. It will be interesting given these findings if insurance companies and future treatment guidelines start to MANDATE the use of chiropractic FIRST – it would be in everyone's best interest!

Chapter 9

Fibromyalgia

Helping patients with fibromyalgia has always been a passion of ours over 21 years. People with fibromyalgia can have a myriad of symptoms throughout their body. Mayo Clinic states that "symptoms can include: widespread musculoskeletal pain accompanied by fatigue, sleep, memory and mood issues. Symptoms often begin after a physical trauma, surgery, infection or significant psychological stress." In other cases, symptoms gradually accumulate over time with no single triggering event. CDC states that the occurrence of fibromyalgia is seven times higher in women than men.

Patients with fibromyalgia are often tender to the touch. If you put your hand on their shoulder, they wince and shy away because they feel so uncomfortable. It affects their mood; their ability to sleep; their energy levels and just about every aspect of their life. Most patients report having undergone extensive testing to determine a diagnosis that explains their symptoms, yet no clear-cut cause is revealed. Until the actual cause of their symptoms is known the correct treatment cannot be initiated.

Fibromyalgia is a multi-factorial disorder which means that there are many contributing causes. Fibromyalgia is oftentimes called a garbage can or rule out diagnosis meaning the patient doesn't have this disease or that disease, therefore, it must be fibromyalgia. Many times, the symptoms are treated with medications that target the brain, releasing "feel good" chemicals (anti-depressants), pain medications, anti-seizure medications and sleeping pills.

The conventional treatment of Fibromyalgia revolves around reducing pain, improving mood and promoting sleep However, the medication doesn't identify the underlying problem that causing these symptoms. These symptoms can be caused by food sensitivities, hormone imbalance, problems with the nervous system, misalignments of the spine, injuries from previous accidents and the negative effects of the undetected nerve damage from which they have never fully recovered.

We have treated patients with fibromyalgia as young as 16 and as old as their mid 80's. Unfortunately, they have all "learned" to live with it, and that breaks our hearts because to be 16 when you're supposed to be your most active and vibrant and be sidelined by constant chronic pain is just horrible. As previously stated, often an accident or injury can trigger the breakdown cycle of the body that leads to Fibromyalgia. For example, a cheerleader who gets tossed up in the air and accidentally dropped but feels okay. One week later she gets into a car accident. The next week her period starts causing several chemical changes in the body due to hormones. Combine all this trauma with eating a lot of junk food and this results in toxicity. Now, suddenly 40 years of age she loses her job and that's the final blow. Despite the accumulation of all the stress and traumas she'd experienced to this point, her body was constantly compensating so she could continue to function and with the final stress, her body hit its breaking point and now she can't even get out of bed.

When a patient like this undergoes our initial consultation, we delve into their history and discover the numerous accidents, injuries and other causative factors which result in breakdown of the body and Fibromyalgia. Based upon our education, knowledge and experience we're looking for any abnormalities related to the spine. Abnormal curvature of the spine produces an undesirable and potentially dangerous effect on the nervous system and the body. So many times, when we're looking at an x-ray, we'll ask a patient "when did you have a car accident?" We'll ask them questions that trigger responses like, "I remember that this injury occurred. Did that have anything to do with what I'm feeling right now?" Patients often come back saying they remembered an incident where they were injured or were able confirm they fell off the changing table when they were little. This allows us to begin to understand why their spine is curved the exact opposite way that it should be.

It's is a wakeup call to most of these people that have Fibromyalgia that they can see part of the cause right on the x-rays. We feel a personal responsibility for every single patient that comes to our clinic to truly get to the bottom of what's causing their health problem. Patients don't realize this issue can be the result of multiple causes or previous injuries that mount up over time. They're thinking, "It just started recently so there must be something I did in the last two weeks. I can't think of anything." We ask a number of questions and really dig into their medical history to solve their problem.

How can a spinal problem possibly contribute to your fibromyalgia symptoms? As with many disorders, especially pain, the nervous system is involved. The nervous system can get affected thorough structural changes in the spinal column. The classic one is the disk bulge producing a painful sciatic nerve. But, there are also other ways to interfere with the function of nervous system.

When viewing the neck from the side, there should be a forward curve with your head above your shoulders, not in front of them. When forward head carriage is present or when there is a reduction in this forward arch, this may cause additional strain to the upper cervical spine or spinal cord, allowing delicate nerves to be compromised. Chiropractic care should improve your posture if this forward head carriage is present.

The upper neck can also be influenced by malalignment/subluxation of the upper vertebrae, such as the atlas. This small bone supports the weight of the skull and is necessary for the great rotational range of motion of the neck.

During neck trauma, the head and neck can be put through a violent range of motion that causes the soft tissues (muscles and ligaments) to tear. Blows to the head, childhood or sports injuries and even poor sleeping posture, can cause the upper neck vertebrae to displace, injuring the soft tissues of the joint. Swelling and inflammation can also be a source of irritation to the nervous system. Scar tissue can develop after trauma, which may affect the precise movements of the upper neck.

The atlas surrounds the spinal cord and as it displaces, it can also pull or tether the spinal cord through attachments of delicate ligaments (dentate). This could cause irritation to the nervous system.

The disorders of poor posture and displaced vertebrae can be assessed through x-rays. Range of motion tests are necessary to see how your function may be affected. In some patients, fibromyalgia symptoms can improve substantially. However, most people will need a comprehensive approach that also incorporates an exercise program and nutritional or weight loss support. Chiropractic care is a natural alternative for those who wish a drug-free and non-invasive approach. It carries few risks of side effects and is balanced by the potential to help patients who also have spinal disorders contributing to their poor health.

That can lead to a feeling of helplessness and not knowing what to do next, which is a common complaint among fibromyalgia (FM) sufferers, and the fact is, many patients with FM simply CAN'T just "…learn to live with it," and need guidance.

One such patient recently presented in such situation. After a detailed history, the chiropractor checked her vital signs, performed a physical exam that included observation, palpation, range of motion, physical performance testing, orthopedic and neurological tests and then sat down to discuss the findings and what specific things chiropractic could offer her. The chiropractor laid out a treatment that consisted of the following:

- Leg length correction: she had a 12mm short right leg, a tipped pelvis with a compensatory curve in the low back. Heel lifts were recommended.

- Foot orthotics: she had flat feet and rolled in ankles that were altering her gait pattern.

- Exercises: she was quite deconditioned (out of shape) and needed help with flexibility, strength and endurance, balance/coordination, and aerobic function.

- Spinal manipulation: She had areas in her spine that were not properly moving, and she had to compensate and use other parts too much, setting up faulty movement habits.

- Nutritional counseling: She was consuming too many glutens (wheat, oats, barley, rice) which can make you feel tire/fatigued/ "wiped out" all the time. She was placed on a strict gluten-free diet and encouraged to use of several nutrients.

They discussed "realistic goals." This was probably the MOST important part for her. She was told NOT to expect a "cure" but rather, a means of "controlling" FM. It was emphasized that expecting "too much" will set her up for disappointment and treatment failure. They discussed ways she could control or minimize the symptoms of FM and what the role of chiropractic played in that management process.

When we can identify the contributing causes of Fibromyalgia for a patient such as food sensitivities causing inflammation, or nutrient deficiencies or previous spinal injuries we are able to help restore the bodies balance and give the patient control over their life again.

Chapter 10

Neuropathy

Neuropathy by definition means the nerves of the body are deprived of oxygen and are dying resulting in a loss of sensation. This can result in the inability to feel their hands or feet at all. The disease process starts out slowly and patients are unaware that it has begun let alone that it is progressing. Patients may mistakenly believe they wore the wrong shoes and that's why their feet were tingling, but five years down the road, now their feet and legs are turning blueish red due to the progression of the disease.

Not only does neuropathy affect the nerves that control sensation, but it also impacts the nerves that control function and movement of the body. Many times, patients come into our office with a walker or a wheelchair and they don't know how the numbness in their feet and their current inability to walk properly are connected because the progression of the neuropathy was so slow and gradual.

Diabetes, Chemotherapy & Neuropathy

Originally, doctors thought that diabetes was the only thing that led to neuropathy. This is no longer the case. Current causes include: metabolic syndrome, certain chemotherapy drugs, most cholesterol lowering medications, some blood pressure medications, infections, repetitive motion injuries, toxic exposure, metabolic problems (including diabetes, obesity, nutrient deficiencies, hormonal imbalances and auto-immune diseases), some genetic diseases and spinal trauma. As two of the ten (to date) board–certified Neuropathic Pain Specialists through the American College of Physical Medicine we studied how neuropathy is on the rise because many different factors can cause this lack of oxygen to the nerves.

Every nerve in the body is composed of two parts: a body (the dendrite) and the arms/legs (the axons); picture a jellyfish. Messages move through the dendrite to the axons and then onto the next nerve cell; this occurs thousands of times in an effort to relay a message from the brain to the body. All the nerves in the body are covered with a substance called myelin (made from fats/cholesterol). Myelin facilitates the transmission of these messages. Any compromise or disruption in the myelin affects the body's ability to feel and function normally. For instance, Multiple Sclerosis (MS) results in damage to the myelin resulting in a patient losing the ability to properly feel and move their arms and/or legs. They might experience tingling, numbness or burning sensations or be completely unable to move a specific body part due to the injury to the nerves.

A specific class of chemotherapy drugs not only kills cancer cells but are so powerful that they also destroy the fragile nerves. The good news is the cancer may be in remission, however, the resulting nerve damage is the next problem the patient needs to address. At Cancer Treatment Centers of America, they employ a similar program co-developed by the Dr. who created the protocol utilized in our clinics. This program permits the chemotherapy to be effective at killing the cancer cells, while simultaneously protecting the delicate nerves. The end product is a healthier post-chemotherapy patient who does not suffer from neuropathy.

One of the biggest causes of neuropathy is a problem called metabolic syndrome. According to the American Heart Association (AHA) metabolic syndrome is a combination of factors that multiply a person's risk for heart disease, diabetes and stroke. These risk factors include: elevated blood sugar (glucose), triglycerides and blood pressure, reduced HDL (good cholesterol) and abdominal obesity. These markers show that a patient's body is building up fat in the arteries which reduces the amount of blood pumped throughout the body (especially to the smallest blood vessels in the hands and feet), accumulating large amounts of sugar in the bloodstream which results in inflammation throughout the body. This excess sugar in the bloodstream not only causes widespread inflammation which further reduces normal blood flow to the entire body but concurrently causes damage to the blood vessels and nerves.

So, what's the solution? Neuropathy, as it relates to chemotherapy, can be minimized. Dr. John Hayes out of Boston wrote a book called <u>Beating Neuropathy</u> and has mentored us and taught us how we can help our patients. There is a three-step approach. Dr. Hayes outlines them in his book and part of it is a metabolic rehabilitation. This rehabilitation involves giving the body the fuel that the nerves need in order to heal in addition to addressing some of the other things that we've talked about in this book and making sure that the spine and the nervous system are working to the best of their ability.

Additionally, there is a therapy used at home by patients that can help the nerves begin to communicate with each other again. This allows the nerves to truly heal versus giving the patient a drug which numbs the discomfort or changes their brain chemistry, so they don't care about their pain. Those drugs have been repeatedly proven to be ineffective in treating the real cause of Neuropathy, but instead only mask the symptoms. Masking the symptoms may result in a patient temporarily "feeling better" while all along their problem is worsening.

We have seen great results from these protocols and treatments. A patient came in and she had had an infection that triggered her neuropathy. The infection had occurred over a year ago, but her health was still declining. It wasn't until we helped her understand how some of her spinal problems were significantly contributing to the neuropathy that we were able to help her. We found she had a problem in her neck and her low back which was compromising the function of the nerves. Compounding the problem was the fact that her nervous system was attacked with this extremely aggressive virus. The virus was gone but the effects of that virus were still lingering in her body and still causing her to breakdown enough to the point where she required a walker and oftentimes a wheelchair.

By identifying the root causes, co-morbidities (the simultaneous presence of two or more chronic diseases or conditions) and engaging her as part of the solution she began to heal. Her personal goal was to be able to drive this amazing car her husband had gotten her. Through strict adherence to the treatment protocol we prescribed, her body began to function, she experienced less pain and more mobility and was able to drive that car! It helps when the patient has a goal, when they have something that they want to work towards.

The good news is that people suffering from Neuropathy don't have to live that way. They don't have to accept that they can't feel their hands or feet, frequently the function can be regained. At our clinic we perform specific tests that help us uncover what is occurring in the body and causing a patient's neuropathy so we can find the best therapies to treat their specific concerns.

Peripheral Neuropathy

Peripheral neuropathy / polyneuritis is a nerve disease involving several underlying medical conditions. It involves nerves lying outside the brain i.e. peripheral nerves, hence called peripheral neuropathy and neuropathy for short. When it involves several nerves, it is called polyneuritis.

Classification and Symptoms:

Neuropathy - nerve damage which involves either a single nerve, several nerves or different types of nerves.

Mononeuropathy - a single nerve is involved.

Mononeuritis multiplex - several separate nerves start to be affected sequentially.

Polyneuropathy - involves several nerve fibers within a nerve regardless of the nerve.

Neuritis - general inflammation of nerve fibers.

Neuropathy may affect sensory, motor or autonomic nerves.

The presenting symptoms are the disabled functions of the respective nerves, which are usually felt by the patient as: Sensory neuropathy

    1. Tingling, burning, crawling sensation

    2. Hypersensitivity to touch

    3. Numbness of hands and feet

    4. Loss of coordination

    5. Hair and nail changes

Motor neuropathy - muscle weakness and atrophy involving symptoms such as muscle aches and paralysis

    Autonomic neuropathy

    1. Irregular blood pressure and heart rate

    2. Bowel habits, defecation, micturition,

    3. sexual disturbances

    4. Abnormal sweating

    5. Unregulated rate of respiration.

Cranial neuropathy - involves cranial nerves interfering with their functions.

Focal neuropathy - affects an area of skin

Causes: The cause are broadly divided into genetic, metabolic, endocrine, inflammatory, nutritional, and medicinal (caused as a side effects of certain medications).

    1. Diabetes mellitus

    2. Chronic renal failure

3. Renal failure

4. Hereditary

5. B12, B1, A, E vitamins deficiency

6. Trauma to a nerve

7. Chemotherapy

8. HIV

9. Diabetic neuropathy - Diabetes is both an important cause and a risk factor for neuropathy. Uncontrolled Diabetes leads to microvasculitis of capillaries of neurons causing their damage. There is an increased risk of infections which have chances of being ignored due to loss of sensation. That is why it is so important to see your chiropractor on a regular and consistent basis to make sure any issues are detected and treated as soon as possible.

Chapter 11

Weight Loss

"Lose weight while you sleep, no exercise required, don't change your eating habits, just take a pill… "We've all seen and heard these claims before and wished they were true. The fact is, it's a simple equation, *burn more calories than you take in.*

The body, like any other machine runs on exact systems and these processes require specific nutrients and power sources to function. Most people are unaware that after they've eaten food, it undergoes eight precise steps to be broken down into a form that the body will use for energy. Our bodies rely on nutrition from three types of macro nutrients: carbohydrates, proteins and good fats. It is the correct balance of these three types of nutrients that gives our bodies the energy to carry us through the day as well as heal and repair.

The process begins with the quality of the food one chooses to eat. In the United States we eat approximately two to three times as many carbohydrates (i.e.-bread, pasta, cookies and cakes, fruits and vegetables) as protein (i.e.-beans, fish, meat, cheese, tofu and eggs) and good fats (i.e.-avocado, olives and olive oil). This imbalance of the nutrients our body needs to take us through our daily routine, heal and repair results in inflammation and a build-up of excess sugar in our blood stream.

This excess sugar can't be taken into the cells of the body and used for energy, so when the body senses the build-up of sugar it sees it as a foreign body or toxin and moves into action to handle the situation. The body will surround any perceived toxin with fat and water to act as a buffer to limit any further damage. This accumulation of fat and water leads to weight gain that will not resound to low calorie dieting because the body won't release the toxins back into the system and poison it (which is what will occur if the fat is broken down).

Why Most Diets Don't Work

Most diets fail because they limit you in either calories or the type of food you consume throughout the process. There's a diet for every craving out there… eat only bacon, eat only potatoes, eat all the soup you want, only drink lemonade… For any real and lasting weight loss to occur the body, like any quality house, has to have a good foundation. Regardless of what or how much you eat, the key component for normal body function is the Nervous System.

The Nervous System has the task of turning on and off each organ (kidneys, stomach, liver, etc.) and gland (adrenal, thyroid, pancreas, etc.) associated with the breakdown, processing and utilization of anything we put in our mouth. If this system has been even slightly impaired by any physical trauma (slips, falls or accidents) it's ability to function properly will be compromised.

This compromise may result in an inability to release the necessary hormones or digestives enzymes to process one's food properly. This incomplete breakdown of food causes the body to be put on alert that something foreign is present and it must be addressed. The body addresses the foreign substance through the above-mentioned method of enveloping it in fat and water and so begins the process of excess body weight accumulation.

When you severely limit calories, as suggested by many diets, your body goes into a state of starvation. This cannibalistic process finds your body consuming its own muscle for energy, as well as, significantly slowing down the metabolism. The metabolism slows down because the body senses that food will be scarce, and it must conserve anything that's eaten. This means that anytime a person on a calorie restricted diet eats any more than they were before, they'll put weight back on because the body still thinks it's being starved.

As you can imagine, this is very physically stressful on the body. Emotional stress also has a negative effect on metabolism. One of the glands involved in metabolism are the adrenal glands. The adrenal glands primary function is to regulate the effects of stress on the body. In order to accomplish their job, the adrenal glands release many hormones, among them is a hormone called Cortisol which is responsible for breaking down fat into sugar. This hormone should be present in the body in smaller quantities for very short periods of time. However, under extreme or prolonged stress, these glands are over worked and must default to handling the most basic functions to keep the body alive. This primal defense by the body shuts down a majority of digestion and metabolism while releasing more Cortisol to fuel the body. Too much Cortisol promotes fat storage by releasing too much sugar into the bloodstream for too long a period; this ultimately gets stored as fat.

Most diets don't work because they are ineffective at addressing all the aspects of the body discussed above. Everybody follows these same principles without exception. In order to effectively lose weight and be healthy one must eat and drink only those foods that are healthy for the body. This means a balance of fresh fruits, vegetables, good fats, protein and limited amounts of complex carbohydrates along with half your body weight in water daily (provided you don't have a kidney problem and were advised otherwise).

How To Achieve Successful Weight Loss

In order to achieve weight loss, there is a multifaceted approach to addressing each of the roadblocks we discussed above. Successful long-lasting weight loss is a lifestyle change. First and foremost, one must look at their eating habits. Changing the things you put into your mouth will have a profound effect on your health. It is always preferred that what you eat has undergone the least amount of change from the time it was harvested to the time it lands on your plate. The more steps a food undergoes before it reaches your mouth, the less nutritive value it tends to have. For instance, pineapple has anti-inflammatory properties when it is consumed right after picking, however, once it has been cut, canned and packed in "natural juices" it contains extra sugar and other additives that not only don't assist, but may interfere with weight loss.

The next thing that needs to be incorporated into weight loss is exercise. Aerobic exercise for 30 minutes daily will help to burn fat because it elevates your heart rate which triggers the body to burn more calories to keep up with the demands being placed on it. This form of exercise can include almost any type of activity from walking to jogging, bicycle riding or even dancing. Weightlifting exercises help build muscle which requires more energy from the body and thus burns more calories than just cardio work alone. The reason being, that muscle burns fat all day while cardio only burns fat while you are actively performing the activity and for a short period after you're done.

One specialized treatment we use in our offices is Vibrational Therapy. This exercise can speed up weight loss because it promotes muscle building in only nine minutes a day. The premise behind Vibrational Therapy is that it fatigues the muscles faster because they're constantly having to combat the movement of the vibrational plate that is the base of the machine. This nine-minute work-out is the equivalent of a thirty-minute work-out on the floor. Vibrational therapy promotes the release of human growth hormone (HGH) which promotes fat loss in the body. It also triggers lymphatic drainage which allows the body to get rid of fat and shuttle it out of your system taking bloating and swelling with it. Additionally, the therapeutic qualities of this machine promote the reduction of excess Cortisol in the body, which contributes to a restoration of normal hormone balance and promotes fat burning and weight loss

One effective way of balancing Cortisol and other hormones related to metabolism is the use of the hCG Program. Many people have heard of hCG (human

Chorionic Gonadotropin) and that it helps jump start your metabolism and ingrain healthy lifestyle habits. This program is medically supervised and lasts for 23 to 40 days and utilizes the ability of hCG to mobilize stored body fat and promote faster breakdown and utilization of this excess fat in your body. Dr. Simeon, a medical doctor from Europe, discovered that pregnant women lacking in nutrition were still able to deliver healthy weight babies due to one of the effects of hCG on their system. hCG allowed them to burn stored body fat for nutrition so the baby could receive the nutrition needed to grow and develop. He began to utilize this same hormone to treat obese patients and found the same burning of stored body fat when he applied a very low-calorie diet (VLCD) and hCG. Patients were losing up to one pound of pure body fat (not muscle which is usually the fuel in a VLCD without hCG) per day. The foods consumed on this program all help to reduce inflammation that irritates the digestive system, joints and causes fatigue. Exercise on this program should involve exactly the same exercise the patient was (or wasn't) performing before starting hCG. Most patients report feeling much more energy, less joint pain and a normalization of their digestive system (including much less cravings, more regular bowel movements and less frequent urination when these are pre-diet issues).

The hCG program doesn't end after losing weight, there is a follow-up phase wherein the patient increases calories while maintaining healthy food choices followed on the hCG plan. This follow-up phase provides a re-setting of a gland in the brain that, among other functions, regulates the amount of food the body requires. This end product of the hCG program helps the patient maintain their newly re-set metabolism, digestion, elimination and energy for as long as they continue to utilize a healthy food program.

If you're not someone who needs to lose more than 20 pounds or you feel that the hCG program is too rigorous for you or you're not a candidate due to health reasons, another way to achieve weight loss is to nutritionally cleanse the body of harmful environmental chemicals. Our body stores chemicals that we come into contact with through air, water, and food instead of allowing them to roam freely throughout our body causing damage. When these chemicals are detected by the body, they're surrounded with fat and water to protect the body from damage. The body does not allow these fat stores to be burned for energy (like the fat from foods we eat) thereby making it almost impossible to rid the body of this extra weight.

The liver and kidneys are responsible for removing chemical impurities from the body. When the liver and kidneys are over worked and unable to keep up with the body's demands, these impurities remain in the blood stream where they can enter cells and cause damage (often resulting in a slowing of the metabolism). To prevent destruction the body surrounds these chemicals with fat (the body cannot burn for fuel) and water. A detox promotes the removal of these impurities while simultaneously eliminating the fat surrounding them; this leads to weight and fat (the kind the body is unable to burn for fuel) loss. Many patients tell us they've tried "fasting" before (whatever their version of "fasting" is) and this does NOT produce the same results as a medically supervised detoxification program.

While hCG is 23-40 days, a detox program, depending on the needs of the patient can last 7-21 days. The programs promote the consumption of specific foods while simultaneously following an exact nutritional program. The amazing by-product of a cleanse is that people do not have cravings because the program provides the body with all the nutrients needed to fuel it for the entire day. Once the body is rid of these stored toxins, the excess fat and water it was retaining disappear, too.

After completing either the seven or twenty-one day cleanse, the digestive system is now more able to handle the body's needs and by following a healthy low sugar diet with healthy amounts of carbohydrates, lean protein and good fats, the patient can maintain their weight/fat loss and continue to lose weight if they desire.

Another successful weight loss tool we utilize in our clinics is Laser-like Lipo machine. This machine works by using a specific wavelength of light that penetrates the fat cells producing small holes that allow the fat to leak out. This procedure can be utilized, unlike exercise, to "spot reduce" specific areas of the body. The treatment is followed by specific exercise to promote burning of the available fat that is now in the bloodstream. In conjunction with the application of a healthy diet, as previously outlined, this creates a permanent removal of this specific fat. This process can be performed as needed.

One of the greatest weapons we provide in the war against those stubborn pounds is our fat burning Lipo injection. It is a specific combination of amino acids, B vitamins and Chromium- all nutrients the body requires for normal metabolism. Adding this treatment to any weight loss program helps keep energy up, promotes fat burning, balances blood sugar (which helps prevent cravings) and improves digestion. These injections are administered two to three times per week in the office.

Any weight loss effort should involve, not only modifying what is eaten, but also, aerobic exercise to increase the heart rate and promote fat burning. Weight training will also benefit anyone who has begun to lose weight. Muscles utilize a lot more calories each day and therefore assist in the weight loss effort, not to mention, change the physique of a person. We recommend that our patients consult a personal trainer who can assess and motivate them throughout their journey to a healthier and stronger body.

It is also essential to ensure your nervous system, organs and glands are functioning to the best of their ability before undertaking any weight loss program. Our staff meticulously evaluates each patient to confirm they are a candidate for our weight loss programs before they ever begin a plan. This individualized attention assures that you will be put on the most successful program for you.

Chapter 12

The Superior Solution; A Three Step Approach

There are three different causes of health problems – chemical toxicity, stressors and physical traumas– so there are three different things that need to be addressed and handled when you're looking at helping a patient. According to the Central Intelligence Agency's (CIA) <u>World Fact Book</u> 2013 the United States ranks 51 in life expectancy. The US is one of the highest-ranking countries in obesity, diabetes and other chronic health problems. The American Institute of Stress defines stress as the non-specific response of the body to any demand for change (whether positive or negative). Prolonged stress leads to hormone imbalances related to the stress glands of the body known as the adrenal glands.

These glands release hormones that control

sleep,

digestion,

weight gain,

estrogen,

progesterone,

testosterone,

allergies,

arthritis,

immunity,

heart function,

fatigue, etc.

The third cause of health problems is nerve damage from trauma. We can have falls and accidents that occurred in the past which can cause undetected and long-lasting damage, not just to muscles, but to nerves as well. Nerves control all functions in the body and if they're not working properly, neither will your body.

Chemical toxicit

There are 82,000 chemicals that can enter your body every week through the air we breathe, the food we eat and water we drink, bathe in and use for cooking. The air is polluted with emissions from industrial and manufacturing companies, burning fossil fuels (cars, trains, planes and shipping vessels) and household and farming chemicals.

Foods contain many chemicals that enhance

flavor,

color,

shelf life,

and freshness.

These chemicals include, but are not limited to:

artificial colors,

flavors,

and preservatives.

Water pollution occurs as a result of agricultural, commercial and residential chemical waste. Fertilizers used in agriculture are found in storm water run-off, hazardous chemical spills from both shipping and industry accidents, Chloride and Fluoride additives into our water supply and improper disposal of medications, detergents and disinfectants all contribute to the contamination of our water. The body's defense against these toxins is to surround them with fat and water to protect against the harmful effects they produce.

Stressors

Who hasn't experienced stress at one time or another? Stress is your body's response to certain situations. There are different levels of stress and how they are handled is a very important part of good health. What is stressful for one person may not be stressful for someone else. Stressors come in many different forms: relationships, finances, work, health and major life changes. Stress is an inevitable part of our lives and is meant to occur for a short period of time to enable survival. Short-term stress triggers the production of protective chemicals and increases activity in immune cells that boost the body's defenses. However, prolonged stress can affect your physical health, your mental health and your behavior. Prolonged stress leads to a condition known as adrenal fatigue, a situation that results in the adrenal glands becoming ineffective at handling the demands of the chronic stress.

Physical

There a multiple cause of physical trauma: slips and falls, motor vehicle or work-related accidents, repetitive stress injuries, sports and even the birth process itself. Slips and falls are a common occurrence in our lives, such as falling off your bicycle or slipping on ice. The Center for Disease Control (CDC) states that falls are the leading cause of non-fatal injuries in children ages 0-19 years of age. The average person in the US will experience five car accidents in their lifetime and nearly 4,000,000 workers each year are seriously injured on the job according to the Occupational Safety & Health Administration (OSHA). Repetitive stress injuries may be caused by work (like a keyboard, or jack hammer operators, truck drivers or high impact power tool users), or sports repetitive tasks.

You Are What You Eat

You would never put sugar water into the gas tank of a high-performance race car and expect to win, yet we as human beings do this all the time by consuming processed foods, sugar and caffeine. Patients arrive at the office with serious health problems such as diabetes, chronic debilitating pain and neuropathy with no idea why this happened to them. Symptoms are the body's way of telling us that something is wrong. As doctors, it is our job to determine the true cause of these symptoms in order to deliver the most effective treatment. Our evaluation includes an assessment of a patient's nutritional state including any deficiencies (Vit. D, B vitamins or an imbalance in the patient's blood sugar) or toxicities. This information is obtained through various lab work and in office testing.

Most people are unaware that the body is 50-65% water. Water has five major functions in the body: distribute essential nutrients to cells such as minerals, vitamins and glucose, remove waste products such as toxins through urine and feces, break down and transport what we eat to all bodily cells, regulate body temperature, lubricate joints and act as a shock absorber for vital organs.

Many people think that if the liquid they're consuming contains water then they're "drinking water". The truth is that to maintain a healthy body you must consume one-half of your body weight in ounces of plain water (H_2O) every day. Most foods and liquids are either acidic ($pH < 7$) or alkaline ($pH > 7$). The cells of the body function best in an alkaline environment. This is because excess acid forming foods and drinks put an enormous strain on your digestive system, liver and kidneys which promotes inflammation in the body. In an effort to balance the body's chemistry it must neutralize this overabundance of acid. This process results in the creation of free radicals (particles that damage cells). Once free radicals are present they set off a domino effect of damage throughout the body that results in poor function or death of the body's cells.

The foods we eat and the liquids we drink directly impact the overall health of the body. Consuming more alkaline foods (vegetables like carrots, celery, cucumbers, broccoli and zucchini) and drinks (green tea, fresh fruit and vegetable juices) promotes a more alkaline environment in the body which results in better cellular function. The typical American consumes too many acid producing animal products like meat, eggs and dairy, and too few alkaline promoting foods like fresh fruits and vegetables. The heavy consumption of processed foods containing white flour and sugar combined with our usage of medications which are acid forming and chemical sweeteners containing Aspartame significantly contribute to the further breakdown of our body.

In the past, the number one drink on planet earth was Coca-Cola which contains 16 grams of sugar in every can. So, it is essential that we really stop and look at what are we putting in our body. No other liquids do for the body what water does. If a person drinks 6 cups of coffee a day then they need to take in half their body weight in water PLUS an additional six cups to make up for the acidity and chemicals that are in the coffee. If a patient only drinks coffee, pop or tea all day and doesn't drink any water that creates a change in the environment of the body that doesn't promote health (one cup of coffee or black tea per day is acceptable). Absorption of a lot of vitamins and minerals is prevented when the body chemistry is too acidic.

The first thing patients tell us when we tell them to drink half their body weight in ounces of water every day is, "I'm going to be in the bathroom all day." We tell them that their kidneys are like a dry sponge right now and they need to over-saturate this sponge to get it to start absorbing and hanging on to water. So in the beginning, yes, you're going to be in the bathroom a lot. However, when a person urinates, ridding the body of that excess water, they are also getting rid of excess toxins and poisons. The remaining toxins and poisons in the body are then diluted thereby decreasing their potential for damage. So, we encourage people to drink a lot of good quality water (alkaline waters like Fiji water or premium spring waters).

Having good chemical balance in the body, like enough calcium and B vitamins is important. There are certain vitamins the body can store and certain vitamins that must come from foods or supplements every single day. If a person eats a lot of fast food and they're a smoker, chances are good they will be very low in essential fats needed to make good cholesterol to help heal your nerves and combat all of the toxins and poisons encountered every day through the air we breathe. The higher quality nutrient rich alkaline foods put into the body the healthier the body is. This makes your body more resilient and able to heal faster.

Oxygen enables the cells of the body to break down food and use it for energy. The body uses that energy to keep us alive; heart beating, brain thinking and kidneys functioning. Four to six minutes without oxygen and the brain and heart cease to function. Our oxygen supply becomes contaminated as a result of the byproducts from the manufacturing industry, automotive emissions and agricultural chemicals. The WHO states that 2.4 million people die each year from causes directly attributable to poor quality air. The health effects caused by air pollution (indoor and outdoor) may include difficulty in breathing, wheezing, coughing, asthma and aggregation of existing respiratory and cardiac conditions.

The body protects you from these toxins by surrounding them with fat and water in an effort to reduce or neutralize their potential to damage your body. This is why it is essential to incorporate a system to reduce or eliminate toxins as part of any comprehensive health program.

Got Stress

Automotive manufacturers recommend specific schedules for car maintenance in an effort to minimize the effects of prolonged usage (stress) on our vehicles. While we can get a new car when and if it breaks down, to date, we are unable to do the same for our body. While stress is present in our everyday life (traffic, deadlines, bills, etc.) chronic unrelenting stress is not beneficial for the body. People don't even know how to relax anymore because they either don't have the money, they don't have the time, or there are too many things going on.

The body's response to stress is to release hormones from the stress handling glands called the adrenal glands. These hormones function to get the body through the immediate crisis and return it back to a state of normal.

Based on the work of world-renowned Hungarian researcher Dr. Hans Selye, when the stressful situation(s) do not resolve, these hormones continue to be released with negative consequences to the body (fatigue, ulcers, high blood pressure, kidney disease, arthritis and even allergic reactions).

The primary functions of the adrenal glands are to control metabolism, balance hormones, normalize blood pressure and heart rate and produce energy.

When incessant demands are placed on these glands, the body's survival instincts supersede these basic functions resulting in warning signs from the body.

The body's reaction that occurs in response to a perceived harmful event, attack or threat to survival is called the "Fight or Flight Response". This response accelerates the action of the heart and lungs, inhibits digestion, dilates blood vessels to the muscles to give the body increased strength and speed in anticipation of fighting or running.

This physiological response, when prolonged, can produce the following symptoms in the body:

weight gain,

exhaustion,

trouble sleeping,

hormone imbalance,

anxiousness,

decreased libido,

mood swings,

depression,

and a weakened ability to infection just to name a few.

"No Pain, No Gain"

We've all heard this mantra, however, but in reality, pain is the "check engine" light of your body. It's a sign that something is wrong. If your check engine light comes on in your car and you ignore it, you'll end up stranded on the side of the road. The same is true of your body, if you ignore your body's warning signs or just somehow cover them up, the problem continues to worsen until you can no longer ignore it.

Every system in the body is controlled by the nervous system. Your heart beating, lungs breathing, your ability to move and sense pain could not occur without the nervous system's control. This is the Master system and without it we would have a very bleak existence.

Slips, falls and accidents produce trauma to not only our muscles and ligaments, but also our nervous system and spine. The body's ability to adapt to stressors often results in a delayed display of the symptoms of an injury. For instance, someone involved in a motor vehicle accident who sustained a whiplash may feel no immediate symptoms because of their body's release of adrenaline (survival mechanism), however, upon x-ray, it is quite evident they've been injured.

For this reason, our evaluation involves a thorough history including a review of past traumas and injuries as this gives us more information regarding the cause of the patient's health problem. That time you rode your bike into a parked car, the falls you sustained while learning to roller-skate, the hundreds of tackles you endured during freshman football and the time you fell off the monkey bars and got the wind knocked out of you all contributed to your current state of health.

These traumas and injuries resulted in damage to your spine and nervous system that until your symptoms began, were undetected, but still present (like a cavity in your teeth). This undetected nerve damage that occurred when you were younger has progressively gotten worse as you've gotten older. When you combine these previous physical stressors with current injuries and other types of stress, the effect is cumulative. This is why when you bend over to pick up you golf tee, your back goes "out". It's not the weight of the tee that caused your pain, it's the earlier traumas you experienced.

Nerves control both our ability to feel sensations and move our body. When nerve damage exists the symptoms produced may show up as too much or too little function (pain vs. numbness or muscle spasm vs. paralysis). A person may experience tight shoulders for years due to undetected nerve damage from a previous car accident and not know the nerves are involved until one day they wake up with excruciating neck and arm pain from sleeping wrong. Upon examination this person may be found to have a cervical disk bulge that is exerting pressure on the nerves that control the feeling in the arms has finally been compromised enough that it results in symptoms. Another patient may present with sciatica (pain down the leg) and be found to have chronic digestive problems as a result of chronic nerve irritation from an old sports injury.

As previously stated, physical stress involves the spine and nervous system. Many people come in and say, "I have pain down my leg. There must be a problem with my nerve there", but what they don't understand is that those nerves start higher up in the back, or neck and are attached to the brain up in the skull. Helping a patient understand that there is a physical component, a pressure on the nerve, a muscle spasm or a bone that's shifted out of place, helps them understand that the site of their pain may not be the source of their pain. For instance, approximately 50% of the people with neuropathy who experience numbness in their hands or feet have been found to show signs of damage to the nerves in their neck or low back.

Evaluation of the source of physical stress (spinal misalignment, muscle spasm, degenerative joint disease or arthritis) is essential in determining the correct treatment. If left unhandled, the body will begin to compensate for these stressors which can cause your body to shift to reduce the stress on the injured area. This can lead to your shoulders being un-even, your head being crooked, or your hips being twisted. This is why you see people with a hunch back, someone who can't straighten up or a person who has to turn their whole body to look to the side.

Now What...

Too often people ignore the pain or symptoms of trouble expressed by their body and believe it will just go away. They ignore it and hope that it will heal itself and that just doesn't happen. Would you do that with your car? We only get one body; we can always get another car. They don't ignore their car but they ignore their body and tell themselves, "I don't want to go in with the doctor."; "I'm afraid"; "It's not a big deal."; "I can tough it out, I'm a guy."

This is the kind of society we live in. We think a little bit of pain is okay, but it's not and it needs to be addressed.

We live in such a go-go-go society. Ironically we charge our cell phones every night, but we don't get good quality sleep. We don't take care of what we put into our bodies as far as eating and drinking and the body is only as good as what you feed it and how much rest you give it. When surveyed, 98% of people in this country say the number one health problem is fatigue or lack of energy. They feel sluggish so they reach for a stimulant like coffee when in reality, water is what they need. Water is H2O and the O is oxygen. The body is in need of more oxygen. By drinking more water not only when sweating and working out but all the time, helps build up a little reserve. Research has shown that driving tired is equivalent to driving intoxicated; that's how impaired the body becomes. But fatigue certainly is something people do not have to live with.

We address chemical toxicity by removing harmful chemicals while improving a patient's nutrition and balancing their biochemistry. This can be done through detoxification, nutritional counseling, oral chelation therapy or many other programs recommended at our office based on a patient's symptoms and exam findings.

There are so many different kinds of stress-related problems that can impact the body. Finding a way to manage emotional stress is essential because the adrenal glands not only help with metabolism but also with the body's ability to fall asleep, stay awake and fight inflammation which then leads into other health problems such as heart disease, diabetes and other conditions which involve metabolism and inflammation. Dr. Dean Ornish, a very well-known cardiologist, conducted research on patients who had severely compromised function of their heart. He was able to help most patients who could reduce their stress but found he was unable to help some people who were "Type A" and just couldn't find a way to de-stress.

There are things individuals can do to reduce stress on their body. Emotional stress tends to be reduced to the degree that the chemical stresses in the body are managed. When the chemical stresses in the body are handled then the other physical stresses can be decreased. We help patients understand why they have trouble shutting down at night so they can go to sleep. Not getting enough rest on a regular basis is like leaving a cell phone unplugged, it never gets recharged and pretty soon it's going to crash. The same is true of the body.

Chronic unrelenting stress is not beneficial to the body and that's why it's essential to have an outlet for stress. Preferably something that involves quieting and relaxing the body and stimulating the brain like reading, crossword puzzles or meditation. Not mindless activities like watching TV.

People tend to eat or overeat when they're stressed which compounds the problems. They are already not digesting food properly (due to the body's reaction to stress) so putting in more food because of feelings of stress makes things worse. Many people usually turn to sugar or chocolate which are empty calories the body doesn't need. This triggers a whole host of other problems including weight gain.

What we eat is something we can control. Maybe the situation causing the stress is out of our control, but we can choose how to manage the stress. The stressor is still going to be there, but it's essential to determine how stress is affecting your body because if you have chronic unrelenting stress it could be negatively affecting the adrenal glands. These glands, and the amount of chemicals they have, are like a savings account. When the chemicals of the adrenal glands become depleted, the body will become extremely compromised, starting with your immune system and metabolism. From there it's going to snowball into other chronic health problems. These glands can be checked and if malfunctioning can be repaired through diet and supplements.

Reducing the stress of all three components is important, but handling the physical stress is critical to patient wellness. For example, if someone has been in a car accident, they've experienced physical trauma but the thing that we don't see is that the physical trauma has caused irritation to their nerves. This creates chemical stress on the body that results in pain and that pain causes the body to release more adrenaline so they can get through the pain and handle the inflammation. That adrenaline output may cause them not to be able to relax and fall asleep or maybe they can't get comfortable, so they never truly shut down and regenerate and rebuild. And then over time they may become snappy, moody or irritable because they're not sleeping and they're in pain. If we only treated their outward symptoms (moodiness and irritability) and didn't address the main problem in their spine caused by the accident the patient's body will never completely heal.

As part of our holistic healthcare, we help patients identify glaring problems that will prevent them from getting well. We look at you as a whole person and not just as a symptom or health condition. At our office we are the solution. When you come in you'll undergo a very thorough examination process to determine if one or more of these three factors is contributing to your health problem(s). Once we determine if we can help you we will review our recommendations regarding the most effective treatment for your condition.

Chapter 13

Your Next Step

Too often people ignore the pain or symptoms of trouble expressed by their body and believe it will just go away. They ignore it and hope that it will heal itself and that just doesn't happen. Would you do that with your car? We only get one body. We can always get another car.

They don't ignore their car, but they ignore their body and tell themselves, "I don't want to go to see the doctor"; "I'm afraid"; "My problem's not a big deal"; "I can tough it out. I'm a guy." This is the kind of society we live in. We think a little bit of pain is okay but it's not and it needs to be addressed.

While people are not going to go to the doctor every time, they get a headache it's important not to hesitate to go when really needed. Some patients have stated their hesitation comes from the fact they believe the doctor is just going to prescribe medication or send them for tests, but they won't really feel much better after going.

Primary care physicians are responsible for handling so many different health problems. They spend their time with patients trying to figure out where they should send them so they can get more help. At our office we **are** the solution, we're a multi-disciplinary office where medical professionals with different specialties evaluate you so you don't have to go to other doctors. Following a thorough evaluation in our office we will discover both the cause and the treatment necessary to correct your health problem.

Unfortunately, we are such a busy society. We want a fix yesterday but it's important to really understand what it takes to keep this machine we call our body running and how to best handle the problems, pains and stresses. Through this book strived to educate and empower people so they understand they no longer have to suffer. They don't have to sit back and continue to suffer because someone's been unable to determine what's going on. You can actually come in and get information and be a part of your solution rather than just feeling like "Oh, everybody I know is tired. Everybody I know has back pain." You only get one body. Once it's gone, it's gone.

We treat our cars better than we treat our body. You can get a new car if it breaks down, but you can't get a new body if it ends up shutting down. Why wait until you end up having something serious like a stroke or cancer to decide to take better care of your body. This is the only one we have so we need to find a way to strike a balance between work and family. There's often not enough time for our family so we put ourselves last. In reality, if we were healthier, we could be better husbands, wives, parents, friends and better workers. We would live a healthier, happier life.

Healthier, happier lives are really what we want not only for the patients but also for the people who read this book. We put this together because there's only a finite amount of things that can happen to the body and there are only a handful of reasons they would happen. It's up to the doctors in whose hands you are putting your life to really help you understand how you got to where you are and exactly what it takes to resolve the situation. The doctors only know what you are telling them. They don't know what you're not telling them. So, they're doing the best they can with the symptoms that you're giving them. However, knowing which questions to ask to pull the symptoms out of the patient is the most crucial thing any doctor or medical personnel can do because only you know what it's like to be in that body. Our goal is to help you get rid of the problem so that the symptoms don't keep coming back.

It's so hard for us to see people come into our clinic that are miserable. We've had patients wheeled into the office, carried in, or they are on so many drugs they couldn't even function and somebody had to bring them in. It breaks our hearts to know that if somebody had understood the warning signs they could have come in sooner for treatment and wouldn't have had to endure all of the suffering.

You may be reading this thinking, "Yeah, I've tried this before and the doctors have said there's nothing you can do about it" or "I talked to my brother and he said, 'Well, that's just how our family is'" or somebody else said, "Oh. That's nothing. I have this and it's 10 times worse." If you know deep down that something just doesn't seem right in your body, we want you to know there is help.

Pain is the last symptom to show up and it's the first thing to go away. Just like thirst, by the time you're thirsty, you're already dehydrated. So, don't let pain run your life. You can run your life. You can understand more about it and take a bigger responsibility for your health.

The whole purpose of this book was to break down the various symptoms and pains many patients feel and share possible causes and solutions to improve health at an office like ours.

We extend to our patients the opportunity to have their friends or family members who are not feeling their best come in at no charge and have a free conversation with us about what might be going on with their health and what, if anything, we might be able to do for them. There is no financial expenditure for them to come and meet us and have a conversation about what's going on with their health. It's an easy way for them to feel what our clinic is like and see if partnering with us on improving their health is something they might be interested in pursuing. We would like to extend this same offer as a gift to you for reading our book.

What's going to happen when you come see us? First, we start with our Superior New Patient Experience.

The Superior New Patient Experience begins with the first phone call where we start a new patient's health history with a series of specific questions related to their reason for visiting our office. When a patient enters our clinics, they're expected and greeted as such. We have already reviewed their health information at our Team Meeting that morning. This is a meeting every staff member attends, on a daily basis, wherein we review in detail every New patient along with monitoring the progress of existing patients. This meeting allows us to problem solve and utilize the entire group to accomplish this task.

A New Patient is greeted, by name, by our receptionist and after providing their driver's license and their health insurance they'd like us to verify, they're shown to a seat in our reception area. The front desk receptionist will personally bring out our brief, but thorough, New Patient paperwork and explain it to the patient. Once they're both satisfied that all questions have been addressed, the patient works on their intake forms while the receptionist prepares the patient's chart and routes their insurance information to our insurance personnel for a complimentary verification of their benefits.

Upon completion of the paperwork, the patient is introduced to our Case Manager. The Case Manager is the staff member who will spend the next few days ensuring the patient is fully educated so they can make an informed decision about their health. They perform a thorough history for the doctors on the patient's first visit. On the second visit, the Case Manager informs both the patient and their spouse about the exact cause (as determined by the doctors) and solutions (s determined by the entire staff) along with any out of pocket expenses they may have (based on their insurance verification) to treat their specific health condition. At the end of the second visit, the patient is asked to provide us with their decision on how they wish to proceed with their care based on the information provided.

Once the patient enters our care, they not only receive a progress examination every twelve visits (or thirty days), but they also undergo several quality control visits to ensure we're meeting their needs and they're progressing. Any concerns the patient originates or challenges the patient may have are addressed on a daily basis at the Team Meetings so as to utilize the knowledge, education and experience of the whole staff and enlighten them as a team on exactly what will be done to address a patient's needs.

If you aren't ready for your own Superior New Patient Experience just yet, or you would like to learn more about how the Three Step Solution can work for you, we have a variety of events each month that are open to the public.

Anyone interested can call our Crystal Lake office at (815) 477-8844 or the Gurnee office at (847) 599-9900 to register for these events.

Those who don't wish to come to an event or are not local but are interested in the expertise we share can visit our page at: https://www.facebook.com/SuperiorHealthGurnee/